LOVE, LOSS, AND LAUGHTER
SEEING ALZHEIMER'S DIFFERENTLY

Photographs and text by Cathy Greenblat

Foreword by
Princess Yasmin Aga Khan

LYONS PRESS
Guilford, Connecticut
An imprint of Globe Pequot Press

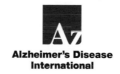

Alzheimer's Disease
International

*Endorsed by ADI
(Alzheimer's Disease International)*

Lyons Press is an imprint of Globe Pequot Press

Text design: Sheryl Kober
Layout artist: Maggie Peterson

Library of Congress Cataloging-in-Publication Data is available on file.

ISBN 978-0-7627-7907-9

Printed in China

10 9 8 7 6 5 4 3 2 1

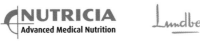 

Thanks to the generous support of Nutricia Advanced Medical Nutrition and Lundbeck Inc., the reach of *Love, Loss, and Laughter* will be greater than I could have dreamed.

DEDICATION

This book is dedicated to all the people living with Alzheimer's and related disorders who allowed me to photograph their experiences of love and laughter and to Kathy Greene, Kerry Mills, and Françoise Guillo-Ben Arous, who taught me by example about extraordinary caregiving.

Photography is so much more than image making, particularly photojournalism and documentary work. There are deeper responsibilities and moral and ethical issues connected to your work when you are given permission to enter people's lives intimately to witness their pain and joy. We photographers become agents of communication, bridging worlds, charged with healing as well as slapping our viewers in the face with information they must know . . . We must learn to make the world a better place by shedding light on dark places but also by providing solutions and hope.

—ED KASHI, PHOTOGRAPHER

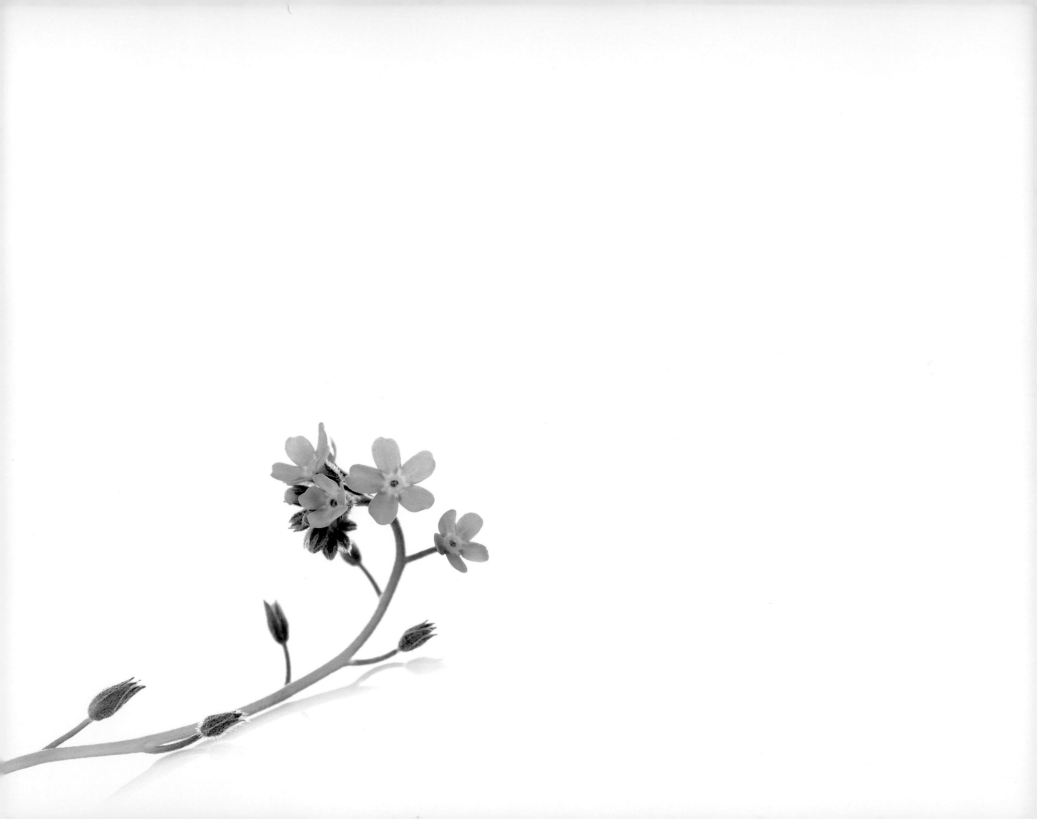

CONTENTS

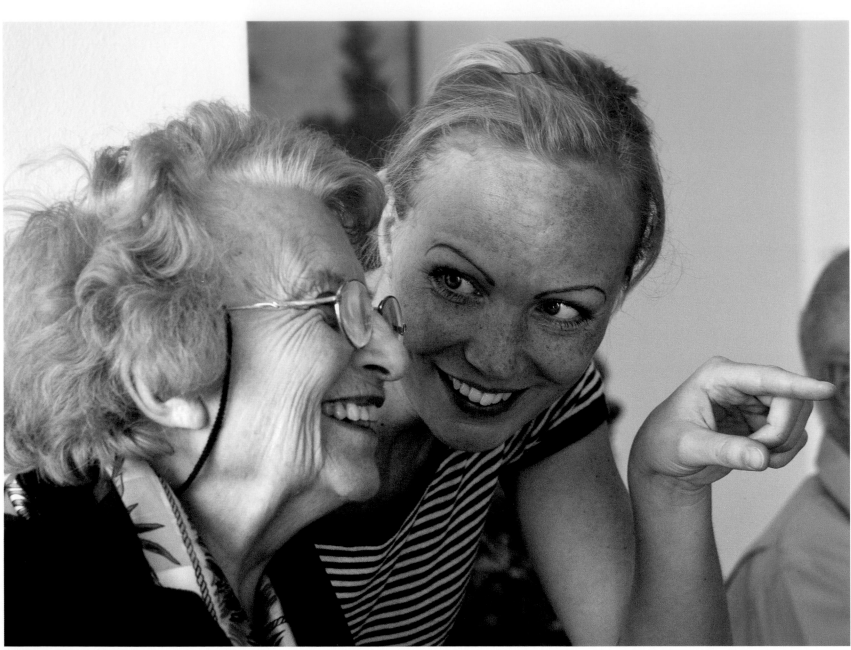

Denise and Signe – France

FOREWORD

I am sure you will agree that this book offers so much more than the beautiful pictures it displays. Through Cathy Greenblat's camera lens and her great ability to describe real stories, we are welcomed into a world that is familiar to many and yet unknown by the world's population in general. We must not forget that dementia knows no geographic boundaries and that behind every case of dementia there is a story and a real person.

This book is not about the difficulties dementia can cause, as some might expect. It is about the lives that continue in spite of it. It really is about seeing Alzheimer's differently.

We have met so many individuals from across the world who are touched in some way by the same issue: dementia. We have been introduced to Maria, who is coming to terms with her impending move, and Len, who struggled to cope with losing his wife to Alzheimer's disease. We have also encountered some great success stories: Mrs. Morimoto, who enjoys singing although she is no longer able to speak clearly; and Anu, who continues to support other caregivers while caring for her own husband.

I hope that you have been as inspired by this book as I have. I know from personal experience that it is easy to feel alone when a close friend or family member is diagnosed with dementia, and this book offers proof that nobody is in this alone. For every person living with dementia there is, or should be, a network of support. This book shows that regardless of where and how you live, there are ways to maintain a good quality of life surrounded by people who care.

On behalf of Alzheimer's Disease International, I am grateful to Cathy for sharing her vision with us and helping to remind us that there are real people behind this disease who continue to live, and often thrive, with dementia.

—PRINCESS YASMIN AGA KHAN,
PRESIDENT, ALZHEIMER'S DISEASE INTERNATIONAL, AND
HONORARY VICE CHAIR OF THE ALZHEIMER'S ASSOCIATION (USA)

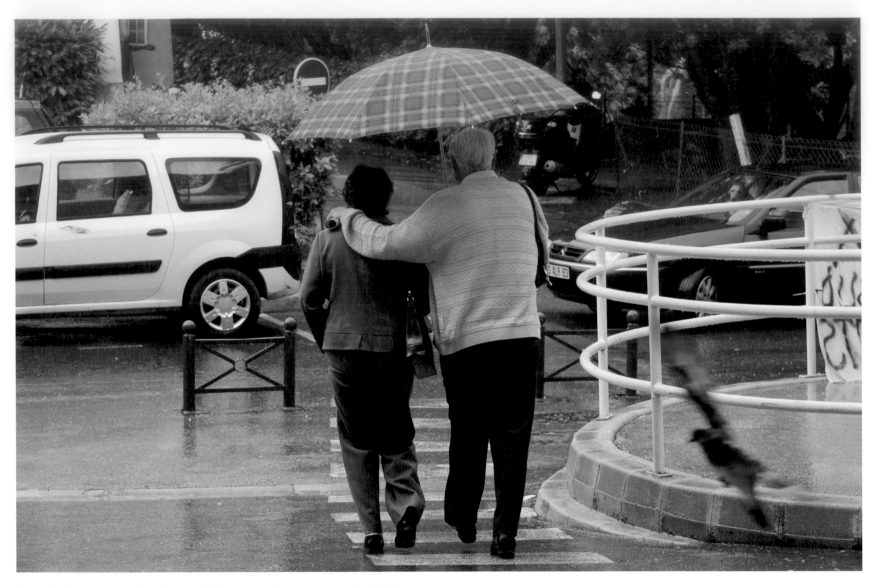

*"An umbrella protects us from the rain. It's important that we create an invisible/
virtual umbrella for those who receive an Alzheimer's diagnosis—an umbrella made of
confirmation, love, care, and true friendship."* —Claudia Bayer-Feldmann, psychologist

CHANGING BRAINS, CHANGING MINDS

I hope that the person who comes into my show and the person who comes out are not quite the same.

—SEBASTIÃO SALGADO, PHOTOGRAPHER

I've changed my mind about Alzheimer's disease. I hope this book will help change yours.

For years I accepted the stereotypical view of people with dementia, one characterized by fear and despair about their changing brains and the consequences of those changes.

What I've seen in homes, day care centers, memory clinics, and residential communities in several countries over the past decade has challenged that mind-set. People living with dementia, along with their families and professional caregivers, offered a much more hopeful vision. They taught me that there are effective strategies for maintaining capacities, independence, and quality of life. It is indeed possible to change what is referred to as "the long good-bye" into "a long hello."

I subsequently read about the paradigm shift underlying this new approach. Sociologist Tom Kitwood pointed the way from a biomedical model to a social model, and others have built upon his writings and work.

This groundbreaking approach calls for viewing and treating dementing illnesses primarily as disabilities. How the individual is affected by the disability is dramatically shaped by quality of care. Enhancement of personhood and efforts to maintain quality of life should be our highest priorities.

I am using *Alzheimer's disease* loosely as an inclusive term, since it is the way most people refer to the full set of disorders. It is more accurate to speak of Alzheimer's and related disorders. And as Peter Whitehouse and Danny George explain in *The Myth of Alzheimer's*, it is imperative to recognize that changes in our brains as we age are brought about by myriad environmental, psychological, biological, medical, social, and cultural factors. Recognizing that complexity is part of the key to changing our minds about Alzheimer's.

It is also crucial to understand that the symptoms observed in people with dementia are not all caused by changes in the brain. Apathy, depression, confrontational behavior, and other symptoms are at least in part the results of responses to the disease and to the person suffering from it. Much of the decline in capacity comes from care practices that further diminish the spirit of the ill person. Patients who are pitied become pitiful; those treated as hopeless lose hope; those treated as helpless become more helpless.

In this book you will see individuals and families across social and economic classes, from several countries, helped to live with their losses through love and laughter. Person-centered care can diminish depression, apathy, agitation, frustration, anger, and guilt for those who suffer and for their caregivers. Despair and anguish can be significantly reduced by treating people as persons, not patients—establishing routines, supporting independence, maintaining dignity, and listening carefully without confronting or challenging. Keeping tasks simple and maintaining and enhancing the capacities that remain are essential.

Providing occasions for humor, laughter, and celebrations of life are also keys to improved quality of life for all.

This approach stresses that it is possible to create and maintain life-giving and life-affirming care built on respect, trust, and love. It benefits those who offer care and those who receive it, physically and spiritually. This model of caring emphasizes the moral aspects of personhood, as well as the physical and mental health of the cared-for and the carer. We can enable people with dementia to fare well—and in so doing, we fare better ourselves.

When I began photographing high-quality dementia care in 2001, I was fearful of the disease and of people living with it. I felt powerless, unable to think of any way to help beyond making donations for research and hoping for a cure. Ten years later, having seen person-centered care and its results, I have a very different point of view. I still make donations to the Alzheimer's Association, and I continue to hope that breakthroughs will soon be announced. But while waiting for that day, I have much less fear, much more understanding, and much more optimism. What I have seen and learned has been empowering.

I hope that these words and images will empower you as well.

True change in the quality of life for people with dementia and their caregivers will only come when there is change at the community and societal level. National dementia plans in place or being developed in Australia, Norway, the Netherlands, the UK, Scotland, France, India, and elsewhere include campaigns to increase understanding and decrease stigma.

The Japanese have adopted one route to a more positive mind-set. They have reframed the term for dementia from a pejorative one (*chi-ho*), which implies that the person with dementia is stupid, to one that emphasizes dementia's medical origins. Now the accepted term is *ninchi-sho*, literally translated as "recognition syndrome." Informed reports suggest that Japanese people are already more willing to consult a physician if they or someone they love shows symptoms of this newly named medical problem, as it creates far less stigma.

A NOTE ON TERMINOLOGY

Dementia is the umbrella term for a number of cognitive changes that usually come with advanced age. It has replaced the earlier term *senility,* which refers to cognitive changes with advanced age. Dementia includes a number of symptoms. The dominant one is memory difficulty beyond the commonly experienced temporary forgetting—why you came into a room, where the car keys are, and so on. It also includes one or several additional cognitive challenges, including attention, problem solving, language, spatial understanding, judgment, and planning. These challenges interfere with reasonable performance of activities of daily living such as jobs, social life, and family life.

Dementia itself is not a disease, but rather a set of symptoms. There are many possible causes of dementia, some of which, such as certain thyroid conditions or vitamin deficiencies, can be treated, bringing about a reversal of the symptoms. Most causes of dementia, however, are degenerative diseases of the brain that cannot yet be prevented or cured. The most common cause is Alzheimer's disease, which accounts for about three-fourths of the cases of dementia. It is a progressive disease that worsens over time. Other examples are Lewy body dementia, Parkinson's dementia, and vascular dementia.

As dementia becomes moderate and then severe, symptoms become more serious. Excessive focus on the late stages blinds us to the many examples of positive functioning at earlier stages, contributing to stigma and fear.

Alzheimer's organizations, hospital and university programs, and other service providers offer considerable help to caregivers, including resource materials, support groups, and training programs. In the back of this book, I offer a short list of resources for further learning.

Some of the best insight comes from a growing number of people with dementia diagnoses who are proactive and are speaking out about their needs, their goals, and how others can best help. They have created support groups, produced resource booklets and DVDs, and spoken at conferences and training programs. DASNI—the Dementia Advocacy and Support Network International—provides an online support service that permits people with dementia to engage in dialogue with others and to learn how to take their place as partners with family and professionals. Heed their words; they have much to teach us about the importance of the emotional, relational, and aesthetic aspects of personal and social well-being. They remind us that being human involves more than memory and cognition.

For now, my goal is to change *your* mind—to help you to see that the person with dementia is still here, and not an empty shell. This book is about living better with a changing brain—whether yours, that of a loved one, or a client. I often remember a Chinese proverb:

I hear and I forget
I see and I remember
I do and I understand.

This book is a journey in recognition: seeing the principles and power of person-centered care in practice; listening to those who live effectively with and even overcome the challenges of Alzheimer's; and ensuring that loved ones and caregivers be provided with the educational resources they need.

Will you join me? Will you incorporate these lessons into your personal and professional lives? I deeply hope that the photos and inspirational messages featured in this book will inspire your journey.

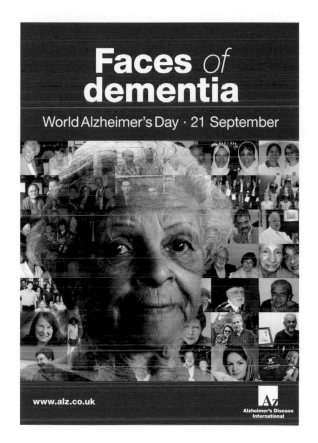

CONTRIBUTORS

The text contributions that accompany my photographs and text come from many of the people who most influenced me, as listed here:

Daisy Acosta, psychiatrist, chair of Alzheimer's Disease International 2009–2012, Santo Domingo, Dominican Republic

Joan Amatniek, neurologist, Alzheimer's researcher, Pennsylvania, USA

Aviva Babins, arts project coordinator, Culture, Arts, and Innovation, Baycrest, Toronto, Canada

Sabine Bährer-Kohler, social scientist, Basel, Switzerland

Cindy Barotte, director, ARTZ Paris (Artists for Alzheimer's), Paris, France

Claudia Bayer-Feldmann, psychologist, former director of the Alzheimer's Association of Munich, Germany

Judy Berry, founder and director, Lakeview Ranch Model Specialized Dementia Care™, Minnesota, USA

Laura Bramly, communications consultant and director, Mindset Memory, Vancouver, BC, Canada

Marcel Brasey, living with the symptoms and diagnosis of dementia, retired businessman, Geneva, Switzerland

Cameron Camp, psychologist, Director of Research, Linda-&-Cameron, Inc., Solon, Ohio, USA

Louanna Cocchiarella, family caregiver, Bloomington, Indiana, USA

Bénédicte Cossève, psychometrician, Nice, France

Heather Davidson, music therapist, Washington DC, USA

Bob DeMarco, founder/editor of The Alzheimer's Reading Room, caregiver, Delray Beach, Florida, USA

Murna Downs, Chair of Dementia Studies, Head of the Bradford Dementia Group, University of Bradford, UK

Hidetoshi Endo, gerontologist, National Center for Geriatrics and Gerontology, Obu City, Japan

Françoise Guillo-Ben Arous, geriatrician, former director of Alzheimer's programs in University Hospital in Nimes and Public Hospital in Uzes, France; New York, New York, USA

Laurence Harmon, lawyer, businessman, blogger-Great Places Inc., Minneapolis, Minnesota, USA

Julian Hughes, psychiatrist and honorary professor of philosophy of aging, Northumbria Healthcare NHS Trust and Newcastle University, Newcastle, UK

Anne-Claude Juillerat Van der Linden, professor of psychology, Geneva, Switzerland

John Killick, poet, writer, Dementia Positive, Edinburgh, Scotland

Daniel Kuhn, community educator, Rainbow Hospice and Palliative Care, Chicago, Illinois, USA

Valerie Lafont, speech therapist, University Hospital Network (CHU), Nice, France

Kerry Mills, president, Engaging Alzheimer's, New York, New York, USA

Sailesh Mishra, founder, Greater Mumbai chapter of ARDSI; president, Silver Inning Foundation, Mumbai, India

Yoshio Miyake, family caregiver, retired geriatrician, Seirin Clinic, and former vice president, Alzheimer's Association Japan, Kyoto

Priyamvada Muddapur, manager, Nightingales Dementia Care, Nightingales Medical Trust, Bangalore, India

Nirmala Narula, founder and former president of the Delhi chapter of ARDSI (Alzheimer's and Related Disorders Society of India), Delhi, India

Marion Nixon, former director of volunteers and of Silverpaws program, Silverado Senior Living, Houston, Texas, USA

Philippe Robert, psychiatrist, director of Alzheimer's service, professor, University of Nice—Sophia Antipolis, Nice, France

Juana Guillermina Rodriguez, social worker, Ministry of Health, Santo Domingo, Dominican Republic

K. Jacob Roy, founder and national chairman, Alzheimer's and Related Disorders Society of India (ARDSI), and chairman-elect, Alzheimer's Disease International (ADI), Kunnamkulum, India

Judith Salerno, Leonard D. Schaeffer Executive Officer, Institute of Medicine of the National Academies, Washington, DC, USA

Loren Shook, CEO, Silverado Senior Living, California, USA

Brahmanand Singh, filmmaker, Mumbai, India

Bianca Stern, director, Culture, Arts, and Innovation, Baycrest, Toronto, Canada

Richard Taylor, living with the symptoms and diagnosis of dementia, retired clinical psychologist, Houston, Texas, USA

Michael Verde, president, Memory Bridge, Chicago, Illinois, USA

Peter Whitehouse, physician, neurologist, University Hospitals Case Medical Center; professor, Case Western Reserve University; director, adult learning, The Intergenerational School, Cleveland, Ohio, USA

Stephen Winner, chief of culture, Silverado Senior Living, California, USA

Marc Wortmann, executive director, Alzheimer's Disease International, London, UK

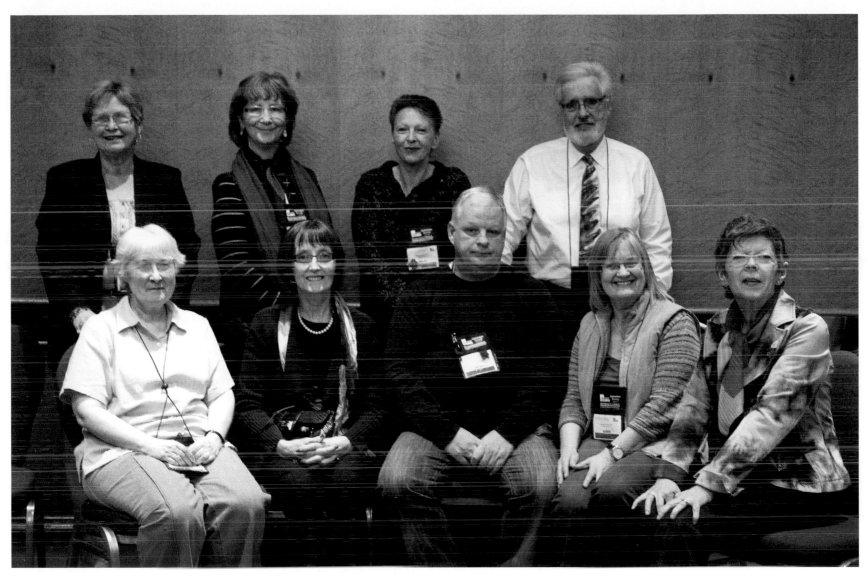

People with dementia actively participated in the 2010 ADI meeting – Canada.
People with dementia took part in the ADI conference, sometimes as speakers or chairs of panels. Back row: Jan Philips, Lynn Jackson, Debbie Browne (accompanying her husband, Graham), Richard Taylor. Front row: Lynda Hogg, Christine Bryden, Graham Browne, Agnes Houston, Helga Rohns.

If you are not a research scientist, you can do little to affect the *disease* aspects of dementia. But we can all take steps to reduce the *dis-ease* associated with physical changes and the neurological breakdowns in the brain. *Dis-ease* stems from breakdowns in relationships that lead to isolation and loneliness, which in turn damage the spirit of those living with dementia. As Michael Verde explains below, we can lead the fight against the *dis-ease*.

PEOPLE WITH DEMENTIA DON'T DISAPPEAR UNLESS WE DISAPPEAR FROM THEM

There is nothing we can do to make an impact on Alzheimer's disease directly, but every one of us can do something to diminish the dis-ease by reconnecting the severed relationships . . . not with a pill, not with technology, but by moving your body, spirit, and heart back into communication with the isolated and lonely person.

The first step that is vital if someone aspires to maintain emotional connections is to know that the person with dementia is not gone. . . . So many messages have created the impression that if people are diagnosed with dementia, they essentially disappear for all emotional purposes—that they are here in body but they're really sort of not here. You hear people say, "My mother's really gone . . ." or "It's just not my father anymore . . ."

The first thing to understand is that this is not true—people with dementia don't ever disappear. There may be facets of their personality that are no longer in evidence; cognitive capacities that they used to have may have disappeared. But what has not changed is that they have emotional needs just as you and I, including the need to be connected to other people. . . .

Ironically, the biggest impediment to communicating with other people is our certainty that they can't communicate meaningfully with us. With that belief in place, we end up acting as if it were true. We either don't come to visit or we try to do things in a pleasant way because we think nothing more is possible, and what Mom or Dad or Grandma or Grandpa says just really doesn't make sense because he or she is gone. With that belief system in place, there is no future for building a bridge. But if we get beyond that belief into a realization that meaningful connections are possible, then a whole world of remarkable opportunities start to present themselves.

—MICHAEL VERDE, PRESIDENT,
MEMORY BRIDGE, CHICAGO, ILLINOIS, USA

Caring for a person with Alzheimer's is often described as a heavy burden. And that is what most articles and documentary films show to the public. What a one-sided view! Thanks to these images we are offered another perspective. We can have fun and laughter, we can slow down our business pace and relax, we can experience minutes of silence and closeness. What a chance for each of us and for society as a whole!

—CLAUDIA BAYER-FELDMANN, PSYCHOLOGIST

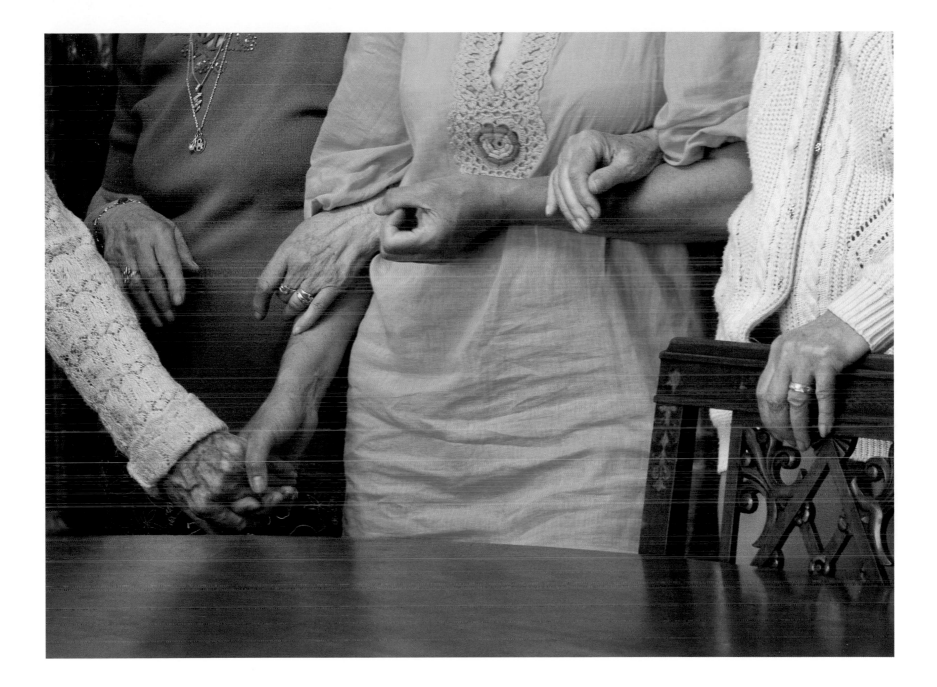

The human spirit in each and every one of us serves as a common bond, uniting us regardless of our ethnic origins, nationality, gender, age, economic status, or religious beliefs. It is also always present regardless of our physical condition or stage in life. That spirit may have been repressed due to circumstances such as overmedication, neglect, or simply a lack of understanding that this is a real person who still feels, loves, and wants to be loved.

All too often people believe that someone with Alzheimer's disease is only an empty shell waiting to die and that the situation is hopeless. We know and must help others to understand that even if the person is unresponsive due to the disease, the flame of their spirit is still intact, waiting to be fanned by the winds of love. We have seen many examples of people responding again, sometimes speaking again after a long silence, when caregivers, pets, and children shower love and affection on them in home care, residential communities, or hospice. We know that without igniting the spirit, medical science alone cannot make the difference. However, when medical science and igniting the spirit work together, the result is akin to magic and the results are irrefutable.

—LOREN SHOOK, FOUNDER AND CEO OF
A GROUP OF ALZHEIMER'S RESIDENTIAL
COMMUNITIES AND HOME CARE SERVICES

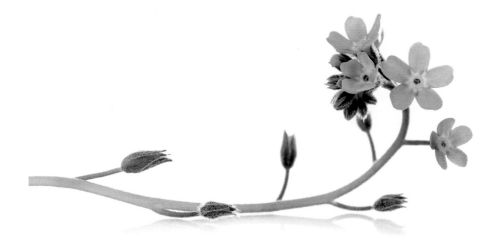

CHAPTER 1

"FACING" ALZHEIMER'S

If you've known one person with Alzheimer's disease . . . you've known one person with Alzheimer's disease. You will meet many here and in subsequent chapters. No one is immune. Women and men, rich and poor, people working in varied positions in industry, the military, academia, and cultural life, as well as those who work at home—all can experience serious neurocognitive disorders. While most are in their sixties or older, early-onset Alzheimer's also affects those in their forties and fifties.

We risk generalizing far too broadly from the one or two people we know or know about. Knowing more than one person with Alzheimer's is important, because there is such variety in background and experience. A richer understanding of this complexity can help us to respond more appropriately, individually and as members of communities.

The common emphasis on the fading of minds and memories—and by implication the fading of identity and personhood—reinforces the association of dementia with permanent tragedy. It also increases feelings of impotence, despair, and defeat—the erroneous conclusion that all we can do is await medical breakthroughs. Recognizing that there is still a person present, though more difficult to reach, we can "face" Alzheimer's differently and more successfully.

As you look at the portraits in this chapter, what questions do you have about the people? What would you ask them if you had the chance? If there is a difference in those two answers, is it something about them or something about *you* that accounts for the difference? Subsequent chapters explore how you can help create a more dementia friendly world for them . . . and for all. You can kindle the spirit of a loved one, patient, client, or friend.

Julian Hughes, a psychiatrist with North Tyneside General Hospital in Newcastle, England, points to the ethical dimensions involved:

Thinking light-headedly about people with dementia is not without significance. To think of them as "shells" or simply as "cognitively impaired" is to fail to grasp what it is to be a person at all. People with dementia live in a context. We (on the outside) can situate them in that context in a way that undermines their personhood—for example, by regarding them as infants or as objects—or we can enhance their sense of self by our interactions.

Indeed, to fail to use our interactions to enhance the standing of the situated self of the person with dementia is exceptionally light-headed, for we are all situated. We are not (after all) on the "outside." As persons we live in the same complex landscape of biology, psychology, history, social intercourse, moral discourse, spiritual concerns, and so on. Their standing as persons is enmeshed with ours; and, if theirs is deficient, ours is deficient, too.

Enhancing selfhood in dementia is a moral imperative.

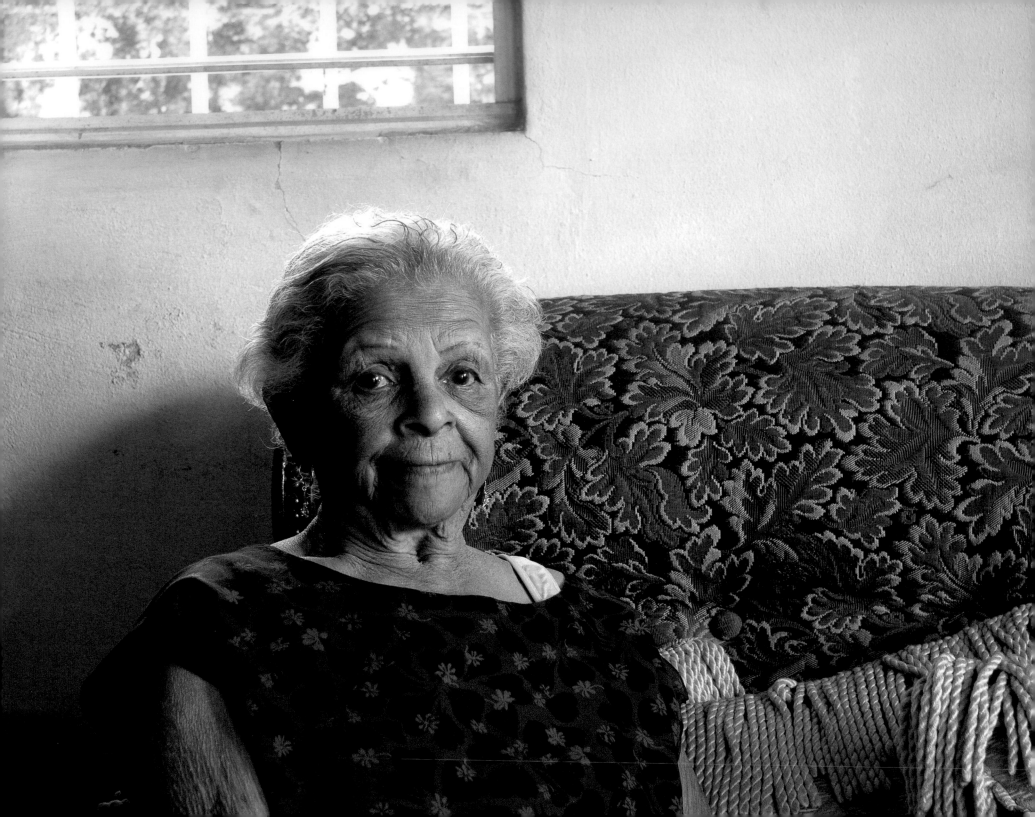

WHAT CARE DO WE WANT TO SEE FOR PEOPLE WITH DEMENTIA?

Care that is directed at the person as a complex and full human being, with human needs and rights, likes and dislikes, different from and similar to ourselves. A person who . . .

- *has had a long full life*
- *has experienced joy and sorrow, ups and downs, and continues to do so*
- *likes to remember the life he's led, who is proud of his life*
- *has regrets but doesn't want to be full of regret*
- *retains a sense of belonging to her family; wants to belong; knows what it is like to belong*
- *likes to be reminded of the good things he has done in life*
- *likes to be reminded that she will be cared for in the way she herself would have cared for others*
- *likes to be reminded that he will be cared for in a way consistent with who he knows himself to be*
- *wants to be seen as a person*
- *wants to engage with the world in a variety of ways—by watching and by doing*
- *is playful and enjoys having a laugh*

—MURNA DOWNS, PROFESSOR OF DEMENTIA STUDIES

Elsa – Dominican Republic

Elsa left school after fourth grade and stayed home helping her mother, not dating and never marrying. Another of her ten siblings was also diagnosed with Alzheimer's, a sister who was outgoing, a professional, married with several children.

Elsa was chosen as the main "face of dementia" on the 2011 World Alzheimer's Day poster and flyer, shown on page xi.

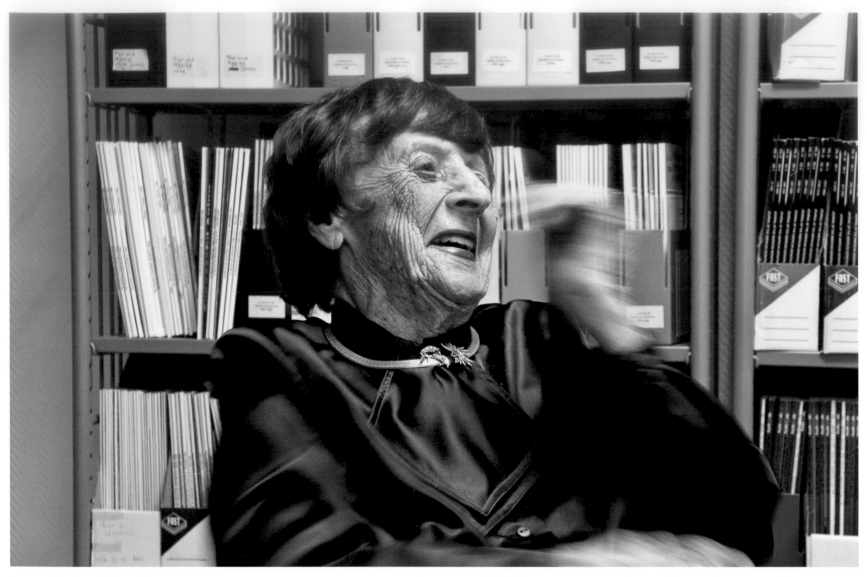

Jacqueline laughing – France

Jacqueline led what she describes as a "golden existence" as the wife of a diplomat. After becoming a widow, she continued to travel extensively and attend receptions. She was considered among the best dressed everywhere she went. Nowadays she seems *untroubled by her symptoms, saying she was always a dreamer. Jacqueline was one of many participants in the reminiscence therapy program in Nice, France, whose relaxed postures and laughter revealed the comfort they developed in a group setting.*

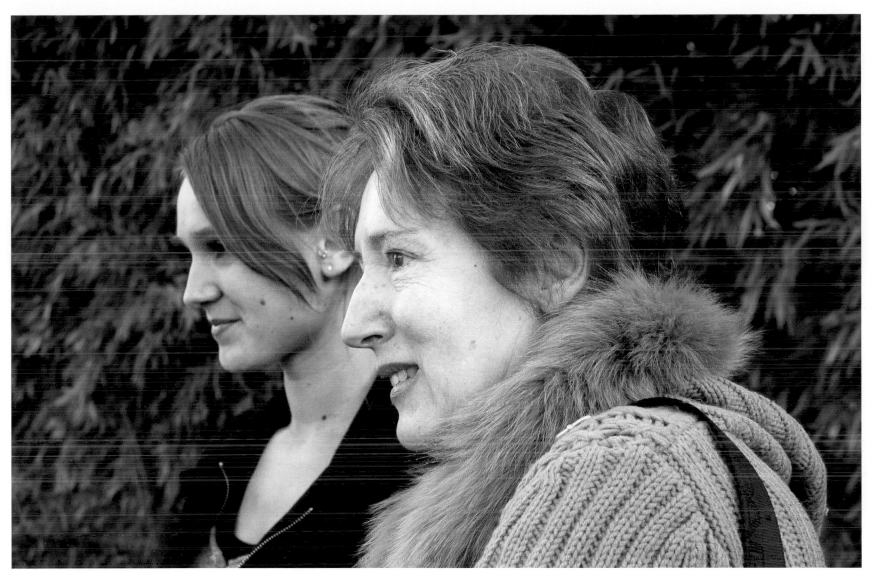

Muriel and Nathalie – France

You may be wondering how this photo relates to Alzheimer's disease. The woman in the foreground seems so young. Perhaps it is her mother who is ill? The answer: Muriel was recently diagnosed with early-onset Alzheimer's. An emergency room nurse, she now finds herself, at fifty-eight, a patient of a different form of care delivery. Muriel is in a research and action program run by the Alzheimer's service (CMRR) in Nice. Here she is accompanied by Nathalie, a psychologist, during an excursion to a local park.

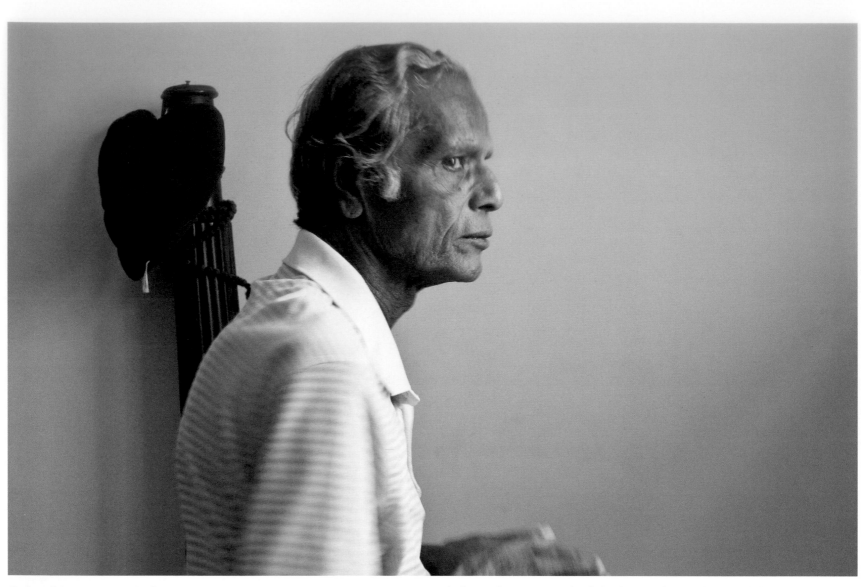

Colonel Srivastava – India

This retired air force colonel has been cared for by his loving wife since a fall that left him unconscious for four days. He was later diagnosed with Alzheimer's disease. The couple moved in with their daughter, as more help with his care was needed. In their bedroom there are many family heirlooms, religious objects, and this pillow, with "I love you" written in German. The colonel walks around the house a lot, seeming to search for something, but he doesn't say what it is.

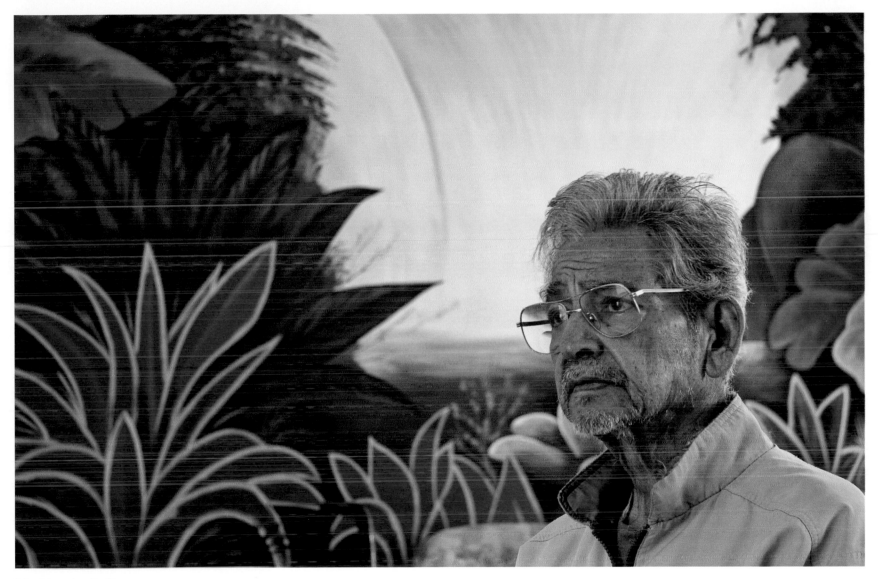

Mr. Noori – India

At the Bangalore Day Care Centre, eighty-year-old Mr. Noori, formerly a top manager in a major industrial company, was saddened to realize that he had less ability to engage in activities that were pleasurable only a short time ago.

Sadness is an emotion, and emotions are life.

—PHILIPPE ROBERT, PSYCHIATRIST

Colonel Srivastava and Mr. Noori, like many patients in early or moderate stages of cognitive difficulties, know that something is terribly wrong—but what is it? Sadness and worries set in. A sense of loss is imminent. Is the answer out there? An urgent need to find that "something" becomes at times the only reason to be alive. Wandering may be an answer for them. Maria understands very well that she is less and less able to care for herself. She is pained at the idea of leaving her longtime home in the barrio, however modest it might be.

When we, as caretakers, understand the emotions underneath the behavior we see, we are able to handle it better.

—DAISY ACOSTA, PSYCHIATRIST

Looking at this photo of a profoundly sad woman who seems resigned to her situation, you feel compelled to say hello to Maria, to make contact with her and at least try to bring a smile back to her face. It is hard to know how to do more without being with her. The ability to empathize with all the facets of the disease is important yet difficult, demanding great sensitivity and personal strength from those who offer assistance.

—SABINE BÄHRER-KOHLER, SOCIAL SCIENTIST

Maria – Dominican Republic

As her cognitive difficulties increase, Maria is finding it harder to remain alone in her small house in the Santo Domingo barrio. She realizes the necessity of moving to a rural area where she has family, but the idea of leaving her home of many years hurts.

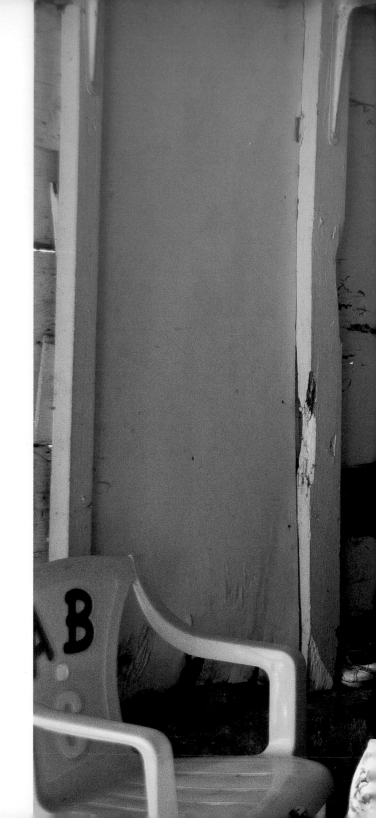

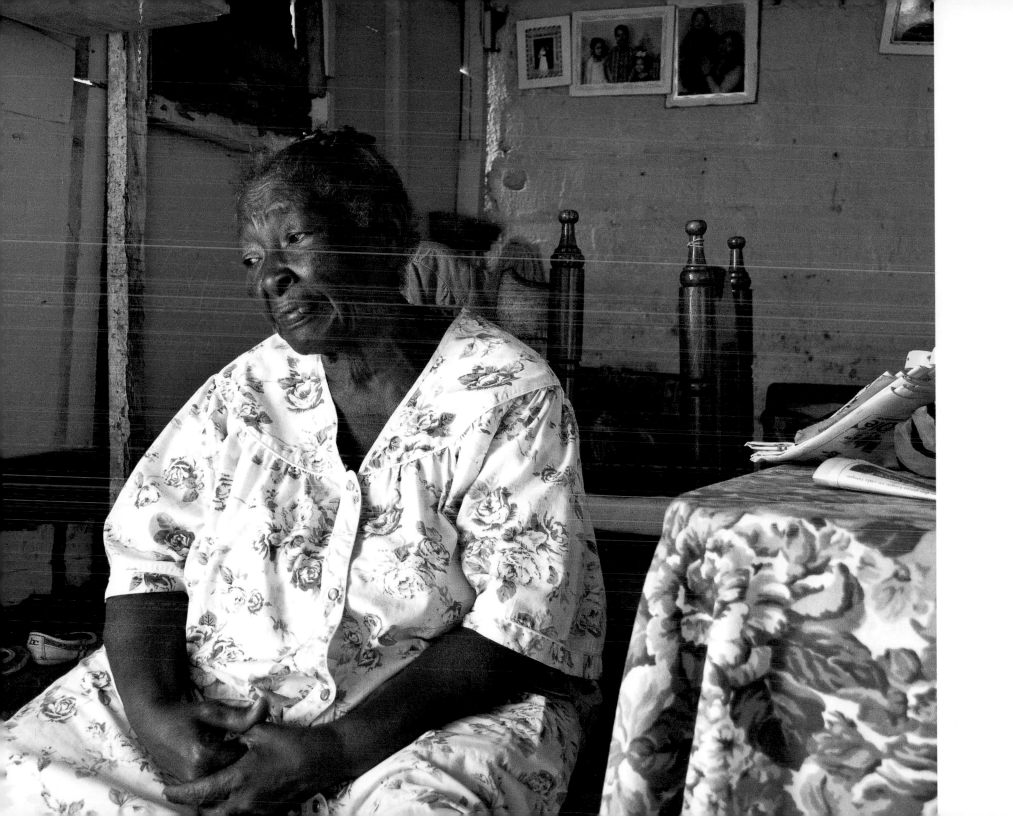

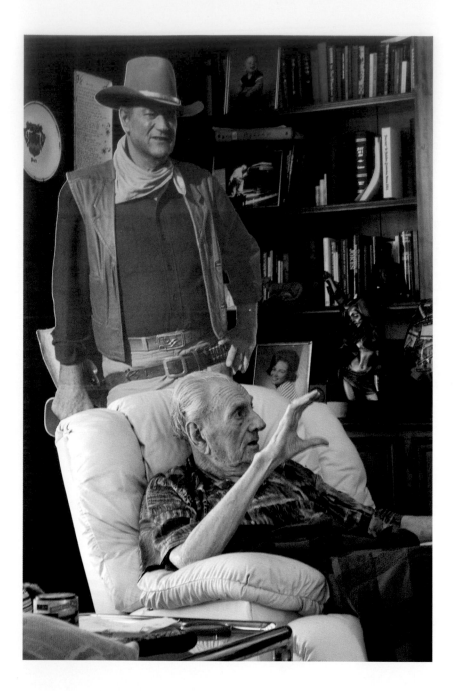

All care programs need to honor the reality of participants by viewing each of them as a *person* as opposed to a *patient*.

—VALERIE LAFONT, SPEECH THERAPIST

Judge Pratt – USA

Judge Pratt developed Alzheimer's disease after a long and successful career in the law. He preferred to remain in his own home, where he lives alone, with the assistance of a full-time caregiver trained in dementia care. His large house is filled with memorabilia, including a collection of gavels and a cardboard image of his friend John Wayne.

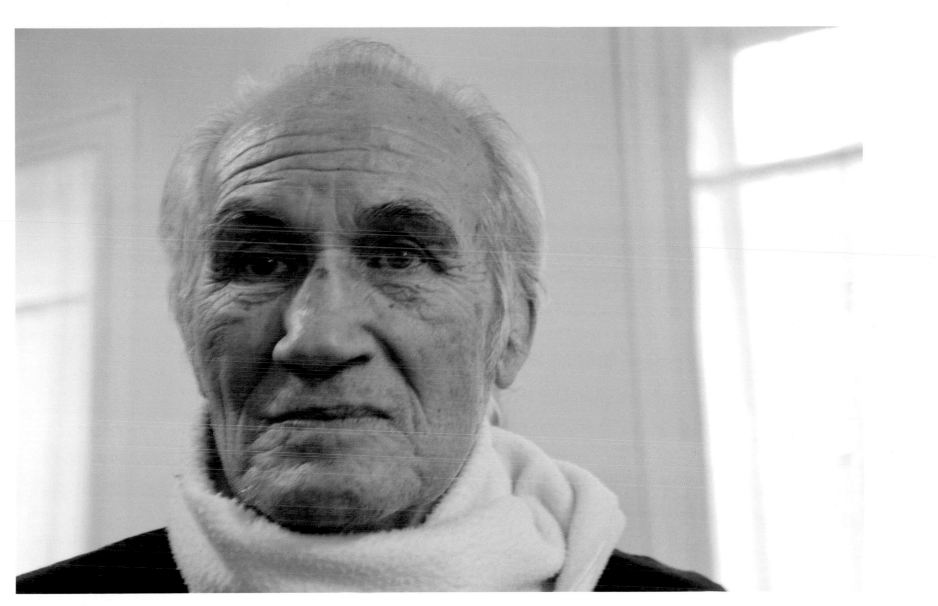

Sauveur – France

Sauveur was a boxer and a cinema actor earlier in his life. Retired, he is a regular participant in the Alzheimer Côte d'Azur (ACA) day program.

In his blog, two books, a DVD, and presentations to lay and professional audiences around the world, Richard Taylor has contributed greatly to a better understanding of what it is like to live with dementia. I am proud to have Richard as a dear friend.

Hello, my name is Richard and I have Alzheimer's disease.

In 2003, after undergoing more than a year of testing everything from my urine to my memory, a neurologist in Houston, Texas, walked into his office, sat down at his desk, stared directly at the desktop, and said to me: "Richard you have dementia, probably of the Alzheimer's type." What he said after those words neither my brother nor my wife nor I can recall. We drove home in silence. As I entered my house, I was overwhelmed with emotion and began to cry hysterically. I ran out into the backyard crying, only to have my wife suggest I should come back into the house, because the neighbors would think she was hitting me. Everyone in my family cried for three weeks. We cried until we no longer had tears to shed, and we were all emotionally exhausted.

The irony—here I was a PhD, a psychologist, with little to no knowledge of dementia, much less "dementia probably of the Alzheimer's type." We were crying for ourselves and we were crying for one another. We were crying for our future, a future turned upside down and inside out . . .

Fast-forward to today. What do I want you to know that only I can know because I have dementia? What do you need to hear from people who live with the disease? I want you to take away one fact about me, and several ideas about how to treat me and others who face the challenges of dementia. I want and need you to help me as my cognitive skills decline. I want you to enable me to hold on to the world for as long as humanly possible.

I want you to know, appreciate, and act as if I am a whole person. That is the fact I hope no one ever forgets. For indeed I am, and will be up to the moment of my death. I am not half full, nor half empty. I never, ever want to hear you say as I sit mute in a wheelchair, lie in bed, or wander around my village, "There is Richard Taylor, only it's really not Richard, it's just Richard's shell. He unfortunately is gone." I am not now, nor will I ever be reduced to existing as a turtle. Just because when you knock on my door, I don't answer, or I answer and I don't know who you are, or you don't recognize me: that does not mean I am anything less than a whole and complete human being.

It is everyone's birthright to live a full, complete, joy-filled, loving, satisfying, purposeful, and purpose-filled life. In other tragedies, for example when someone loses a leg, their family, the community, the government, and the world rally around them and seek to provide a prosthetic leg. When a human being is losing the ability to control some of her or his cognitive functions, the family cries, the community draws away, the governments are too busy saving their banking systems . . .

I believe professionals and, to a lesser degree, carers have an obligation to do more than love us, or like us, or be kind to us. Of course, we want and need this—but everyone wants and needs love in their lives. It is the way everyone wants to be treated, to be respected, to be loved, to be honored for being themselves.

—RICHARD TAYLOR, CLINICAL PSYCHOLOGIST;
PERSON LIVING WITH THE SYMPTOMS AND DIAGNOSIS OF DEMENTIA

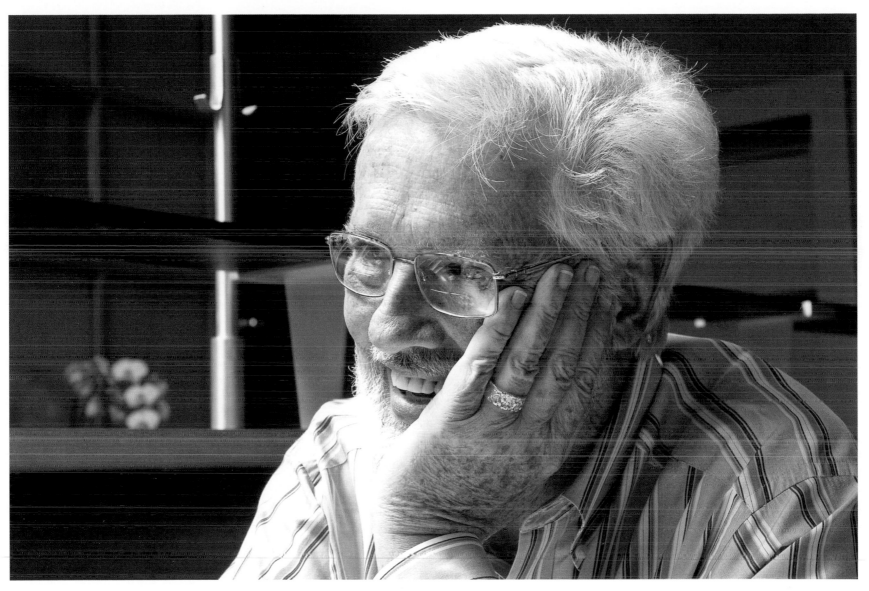

Richard Taylor in Washington, DC – USA

"I have a large vocabulary, a loud voice, and a PhD—a great combination if one is trying to hide one's early-onset Alzheimer's disease."

There are a great many publications to help individuals and family caregivers find a better way of living with a dementia diagnosis. These include blogs such as Bob DeMarco's Alzheimer's Reading Room, memoirs by caregivers recounting their experiences, practical guides by Alzheimer's associations and other organizations, and books, articles, and blogs by people with dementia including Richard Taylor, Christine Bryden, James McKillop, and Marcel Brasey. There are also many volumes by professionals, a few of which are listed in the resources section at the back of this book.

While many people suspect that they or a loved one is experiencing cognitive difficulties that are more serious than normal brain aging, they hesitate to see a doctor until the symptoms are far advanced. The problem is exacerbated by the fact that many doctors are not knowledgeable about the topic, or they hesitate to inform people of their diagnosis. Murna Downs, professor with the Bradford Dementia Group at the University of Bradford in the United Kingdom, advises patients, family members, and physicians as follows:

People need to be told in a sensitive manner that they have a progressive brain disease that results in cognitive impairment. They need to be told that they must adapt their lives to live with this impairment and that there are interventions (such as cognitive rehabilitation) and psychosocial supports (such as support groups) available to help them adjust.

Having assisted many individual patients, and having created excellent day and residential programs in southern France, geriatrician and former director of Alzheimer's programs in Nimes and Uzes, France, Françoise Guillo-Ben Arous highlights the multiple problems that must be addressed over time:

Different deficits often accompany the cognitive handicaps of people with dementia. Pains, trouble walking, joint diseases, respiratory or cardiac difficulties, loss of vision or hearing . . . all of these compromise the autonomy of patients suffering from problems of memory and orientation. Getting up and walking alone require a considerable effort, particularly if the environment is not well adapted for them.

Their quality of life can be changed significantly by care that takes such deficits seriously into account—for example, by providing glasses and hearing aids for those who need them—but also by modifying the architectural design and interior of private homes, day-care centers, and residential facilities.

A series of guides, "By Us for Us," is produced by the Murray Alzheimer Research and Education Program in Waterloo, Canada (see the resources section). Their advice on daily living includes ideas about finances, safety and security, minimizing stress, visual cues, developing routines, entertaining, and electronic aids, and these general suggestions for people with Alzheimer's:

- Keep life simple.
- Keep your sense of humor.
- Plan ahead.
- Communicate your needs to your partner, friends, and family; ask for and accept help.
- Don't be ashamed—talk openly about your disease.
- Check out transportation resources in your own community, including organizations that offer volunteer drivers for medical appointments and grocery shopping.
- Stay engaged—for example, volunteer in your community.
- Attend a support group.
- Create a memory box and start writing or taping your life story—this is a good way to share with others what is meaningful to you and what you want them to know about you.

FACING ALZHEIMER'S AT THE SOCIETAL LEVEL

To spread Alzheimer's Disease International's (ADI's) vision of an improved quality of life for people with dementia and their families throughout the world, there are major obstacles to overcome:

- lack of sufficient support for individuals and family caregivers
- absence of systematic screenings
- shortage of doctors trained in gerontology
- reluctance of general practitioners to announce diagnoses even when they know how to make them
- insufficient numbers of memory clinics and day programs
- limited training opportunities for family members and professionals
- high costs for residential care
- excessive use of pharmacological "solutions" for difficult behavior
- ageism and stigmas about Alzheimer's disease

A more dementia-friendly world requires major improvements in public awareness accessibility and responsiveness by health/social service systems.

Figures in ADI's World Alzheimer's Report 2009 indicate that dementia will be a major problem throughout the world in coming decades. The main challenge is the growth in sheer numbers of people with dementia in developing countries such as India and China. The challenge for organizations like ADI is to find ways to support these countries while understanding their cultural differences. Although there has been a good deal of progress in clinical research toward better treatments, the results should directly benefit family caregivers. Collaborative efforts between ADI and the World Health Organization must advocate for lower treatment and care costs and fees.

Hearing the stories of individuals with dementia and their caregivers is vital to our understanding. One of the most memorable ADI conference events took place in New Zealand (2001), when Christine Bryden came forward as the first person with dementia to speak during a keynote session. She gave a candid and inspiring account of living with dementia. Her passionate speech received a standing ovation from a packed audience. A man shared the story of his life with the disease at the Kyoto conference in 2004. He was the first person from Japan to do so at a public conference, overcoming many difficulties and linguistic barriers. It was a remarkable breakthrough, because dementia had been looked upon as a taboo in Japan.

—YOSHIO MIYAKE, GERIATRICIAN

People with early-onset Alzheimer's disease tend to be the forgotten few when it comes to the disease and obtaining services. Such services and most of the funding for families dealing with dementia tend to be reserved for people over the age of sixty-five. In addition, the family must deal with a lost income and a partner who cannot contribute as much physically or emotionally to the family unit. Can you imagine if you were a busy mother, working, driving kids around, volunteering, involved with friends and community, and then, suddenly, you were unable to do any of that? How would that affect you? Your children? Your spouse? Your extended family? The impact is staggering. We must do a better job of recognizing the existence of people with early-onset Alzheimer's disease.

—LAURA BRAMLY, COMMUNICATIONS CONSULTANT

Celebrating is essential. Don't miss any occasion.

Celebrate the pleasure of being together, at the beginning of spring or summer, when cherry blossoms appear or the first snow comes, on Passover, Easter, Christmas, the end of Ramadan, Memorial Day, or Independence Day . . . Find the inspiration and use the occasion of a special moment to celebrate. Birthdays, anniversaries, public or religious holidays, national and historical days are all in our collective memory, and these dates are times to sing joyfully about the rhythms of life or the year.

Celebrating creates the state of mind in which you are able to feel and perceive the very special moments of the event. You can do it with just you and your beloved or just a few friends, at home, on a picnic, or during a short visit to a museum or downtown.

Celebrating should become part of the culture of institutions that treat patients with Alzheimer's. Organize and seek help from the administrators. You will need a plan, and additional material support. Invite musicians and artists. If you plan an excursion, ensure transport and access, and secure the path. Don't be too ambitious; patients can tire easily.

Prepare to be happy. Prepare also to be exhausted afterward, but oh so satisfied! You will have much more work than on other days. But the quality of life for family and friends, for patients and staff, will improve greatly. Celebrating with laughter and music is therapeutic.

—FRANÇOISE GUILLO-BEN AROUS, GERIATRICIAN

CHAPTER 2

CELEBRATING LIFE

Everyone knows about the losses that Alzheimer's and related disorders bring, but few people realize that joy can continue. Playfulness and laughter emerge from a variety of sources, including parties, interactions built on smiles and humor, and LaughterYoga.

People with Alzheimer's are less apathetic, agitated, and anxious when they have an opportunity to participate in activities that evoke positive emotions. And those around them can rejoice in seeing their joy. This should inspire us to create richer experiences more frequently. Dr. Madan Kataria, founder of LaughterYoga, said it so well: "Don't leave laughter to chance. Make a commitment from within and go for it." Remember, too, that life is also celebrated through moments of quiet joy, alone or together. Finding or creating such moments is essential. Make a commitment and go for it.

Richard Taylor, himself a person with Alzheimer's, addresses the power of laughter:

Laughter is not a key to slowing the progress of the symptoms of Alzheimer's or any other form of dementia. Laughter is not a key to curing any form of dementia. Laughter can even have a hard and hurtful edge to it when it is not shared by everyone in the room.

On the other hand, laughter can break the tension of a moment. Laughter can transform lemons into lemonade, if only for a moment or two. Laughter can, temporarily at least, heal the nicks and cuts to the self-esteem, the loss of self-control, and the purposeless lives of too many folks who live with ever-increasing symptoms of dementia.

Laughter is glue that can hold couples together in the most stressful of moments. On one of the first days after my diagnosis, there was a moment of absurdity in our household, and I started to laugh. My wife, Linda, then started to laugh. We sat there laughing until we cried tears of joy, tears that connected us, tears that proved we were going to get through "this," whatever this was going to turn out to be, to get through it together, loving each other, laughing at ourselves and with each other.

Laughter is a common denominator of our humanity. Laughter, intense laughing, is what separates humans from all other forms of life on our planet. Animals can be happy, but they cannot laugh out loud, laugh until they cry or until their sides hurt. People living with dementia can laugh that hard. Unfortunately they seldom do. We should share, encourage, and point out all moments of joy and glee to one another, especially to people living with dementia whose lives are too much defined by sadness. Laughter can reinforce the joy, the purposefulness, the connectedness of all human beings if only we can see the forest of humanity instead of the trees of dementia.

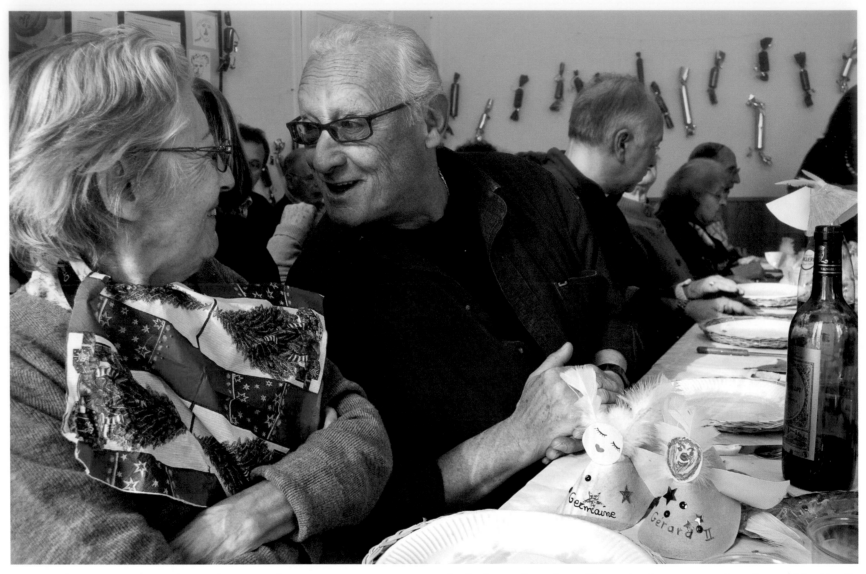

Gerard, day-care program driver, flirting with Germaine – France

Germaine has long moments of confusion, but she was fully centered during an extended exchange with Gerard at the Alzheimer's Côte d'Azur Christmas party. He put their place markers together and charmed her with flirtatious behavior, based on having known Germaine and her mother for many years. Later he passed her his cell phone and urged her to "call Santa Claus and tell him what you want for Christmas." He added, "What I want is more time with you." Germaine giggled, took the phone, and played along with a big smile.

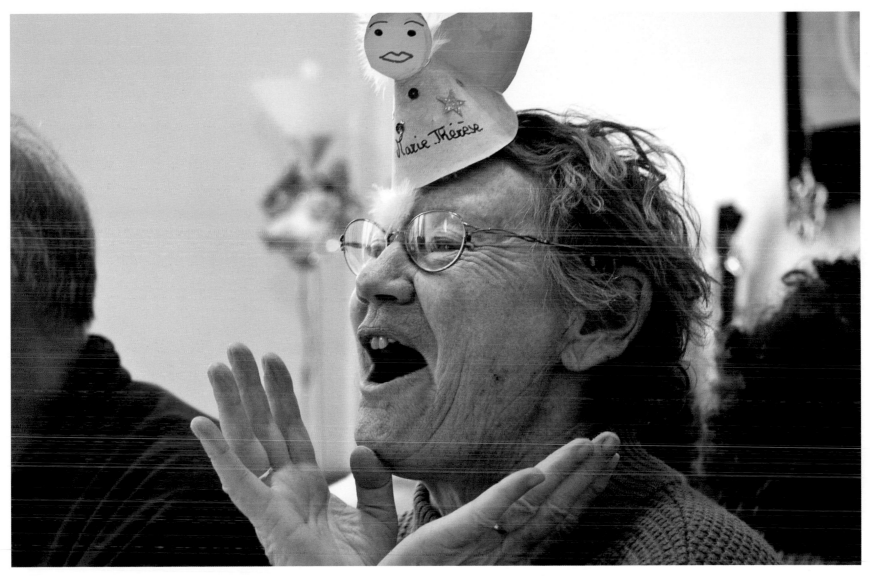

Marie-Therese at the ACA Christmas party – France

Marie-Therese is sensitive and emotional and sometimes alternates between tears and laughter in a short time span. Her laughter is more frequent, however. "It's what my mother taught me," she explained, "and it's the outlook I had when working as a midwife." Widowed and now living in a retirement home, she comes to the Alzheimer's Côte d'Azur day program three days a week as one of their most committed participants.

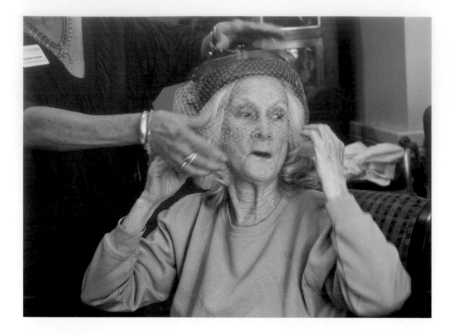

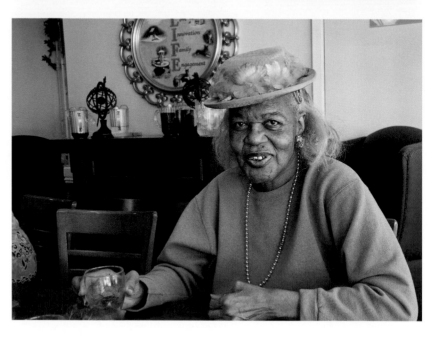

"The Luncheon" at Silverado, Kingwood – USA

Six women at this residential Alzheimer's community in Texas were taken by staff members to a flea market to select and purchase hats. The next day, a special table was set for them in the dining room. Each woman arrived sporting her new hat.

At one point Jerre asked if I liked her black hat. When I said that I did, she replied, "It's a little crazy and off balance, just like me!" We both laughed.

At the end of the luncheon, Lois charmed Sabrina, the daughter of a staff member, by placing her hat on Sabrina's head. Everyone had a good time.

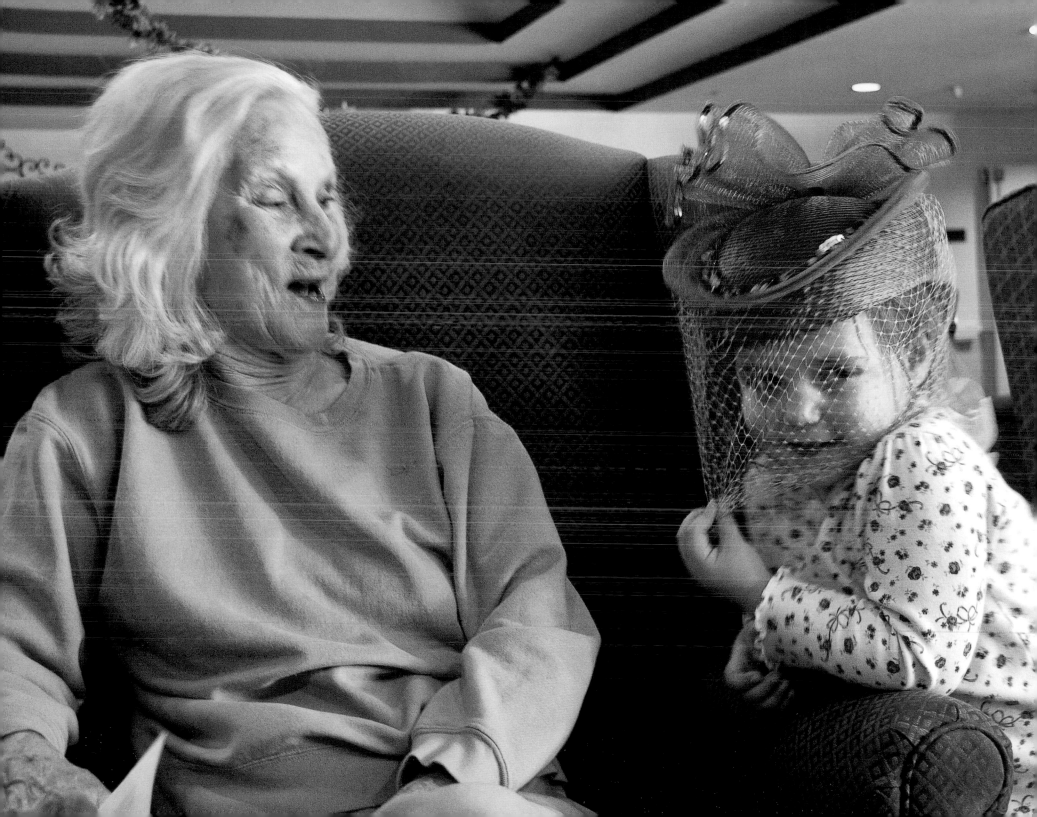

What a great party! Forget about sadness! It is wonderful to share moments of joy and fun. The children, residents, and staff members celebrating together seem to be like a big family, and there is no one complaining about the flour on their cheeks or on the floor. That's what makes us feel at home.

—CLAUDIA BAYER-FELDMANN, PSYCHOLOGIST

The Hajyodo party – Japan

At this party, organized by the staff at a nine-resident group home in Hajyodo, decorations were put up and candies were buried in trays of flour. One by one, several of the residents, each with a hat on backward to protect her hair, "bobbed" for the candies, picking them up in her teeth. Many staff members did the same thing. The result was usually a face covered with flour. After being shown how they looked in a mirror, they were then photographed by a staff member. Finally, staff members with flour-covered faces kissed those who had not bobbed for the candy. The whole event was full of laughter.

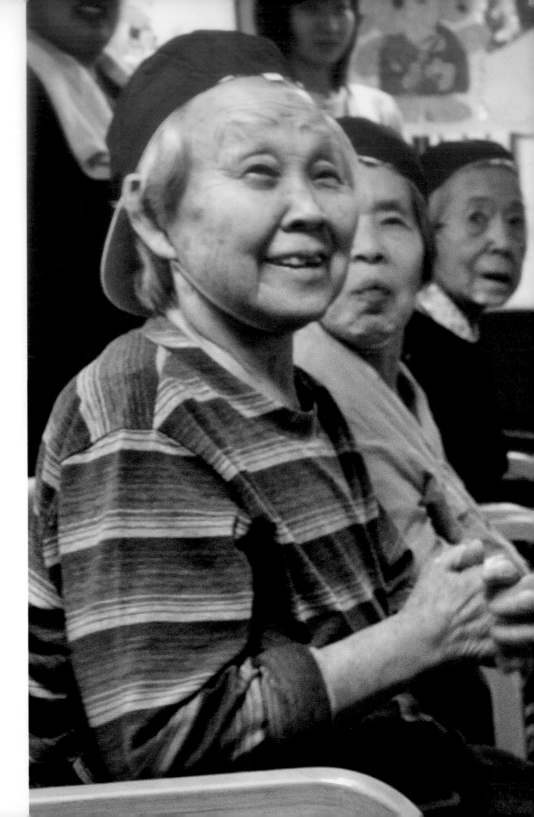

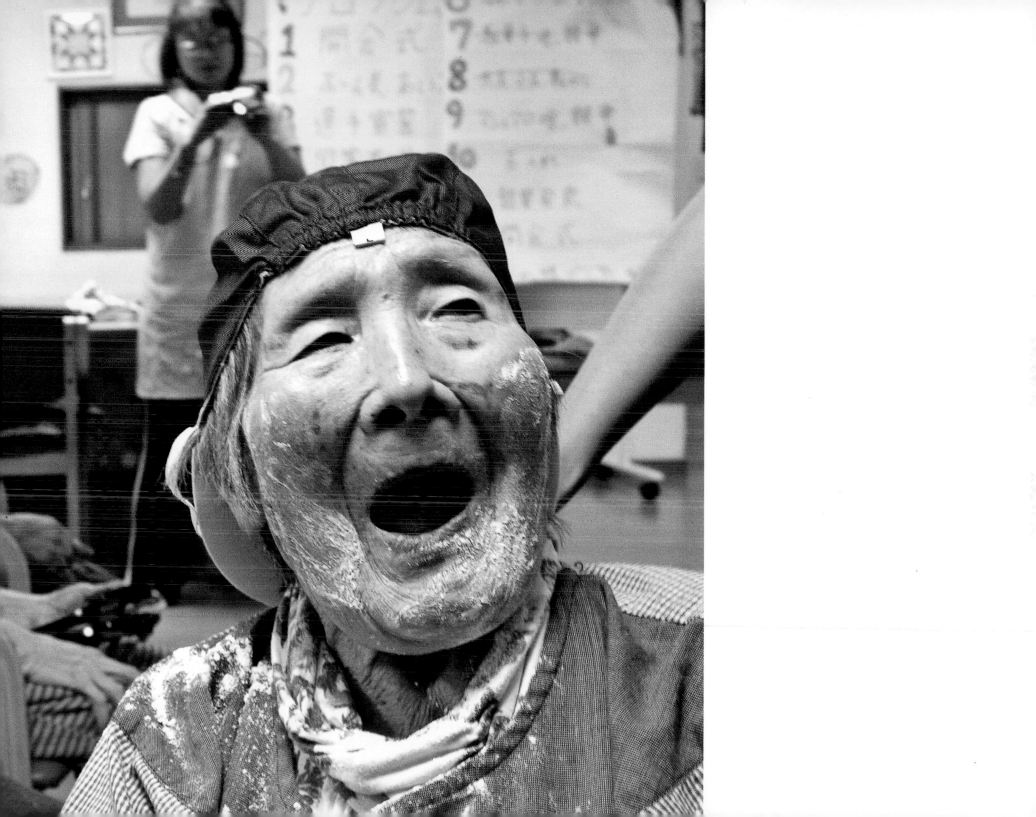

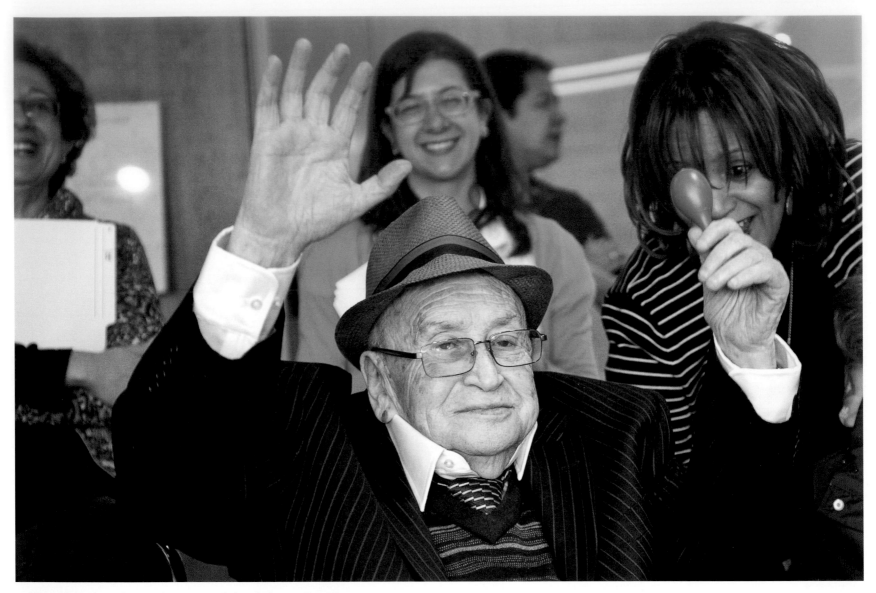

Andy celebrating his eighty-seventh birthday – Canada

We should always remember that people with dementia are not "children" and should not be treated as if they have reverted to childhood. Like other adults, though, they can love things children love, such as a birthday celebration.

Located in Toronto, Canada, Baycrest is a world-premier academic health science center focused on aging. Activity directors and other visitors from around the world are inspired by seeing how much can be done to celebrate life.

At Baycrest, the Department of Culture, Arts, and Innovation works in partnership with staff across the center to develop programs that focus on engaging elders in meaningful cultural, spiritual, and arts-based activities. We believe that this kind of involvement is vital to health, well-being, and overall quality of life.

A meaningful and familiar context is purposefully created to support participation by the residents with dementia.

Celebrating life within the Baycrest environment includes holiday events; birthday gatherings; family days; weekly concerts; intergenerational programs; art talks; glee club; museum on wheels; music, dance, and art; cultural outings; social teas; gardening clubs; drumming circles; and much more.

Program planning involves everyone. By creating environments that are alive, dynamic, and relationship-centered, these programs invite residents, families, volunteers, and staff to come together in community.

—AVIVA BABINS AND BIANCA STERN,
CULTURE AND ARTS PROGRAM SPECIALISTS

What a great experience this was. Elsie had on her disagreeable face as we started. It's the face my mother wore when she was unsure of the whole situation and wanted to hide her uncertainty and vulnerability behind a facade of distaste. As the session progressed, Elsie started to get more and more into it, and she attempted some of the actions and sounds along with everyone else.

Then Jody started the "Amazing" exercise. Part of LaughterYoga is affirmation . . . affirming the value of each person in the room as a person with something important to contribute. When I went around to Elsie, not only did she do the pointing, but she yelled, and I mean yelled, "I'M AMAZING, YOU'RE AMAZING, WE'RE AMAZING!" Wow.

—LAURA BRAMLY, COMMUNICATIONS CONSULTANT

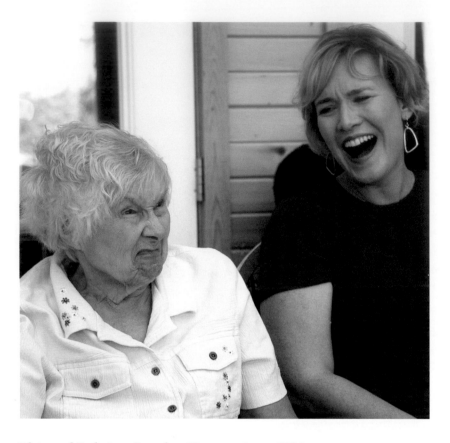

Elsie and Jody in a LaughterYoga session – USA

*I first experienced LaughterYoga in Mumbai. There a group between the ages of forty-five and eighty-five showed how this combination of physical exercises, breathing exercises, and minimal verbal communication was **fun**! Seeking further information, I met with the originator, Dr. Madan Kataria, in Bangalore a few days later.*

*In these photos Jody Ross, a LaughterYoga teacher in the United States, interacts with a group with dementia. Elsie reluctantly agreed to participate, making it clear that she would **not** have a good time. She was transformed into an active and enthusiastic participant.*

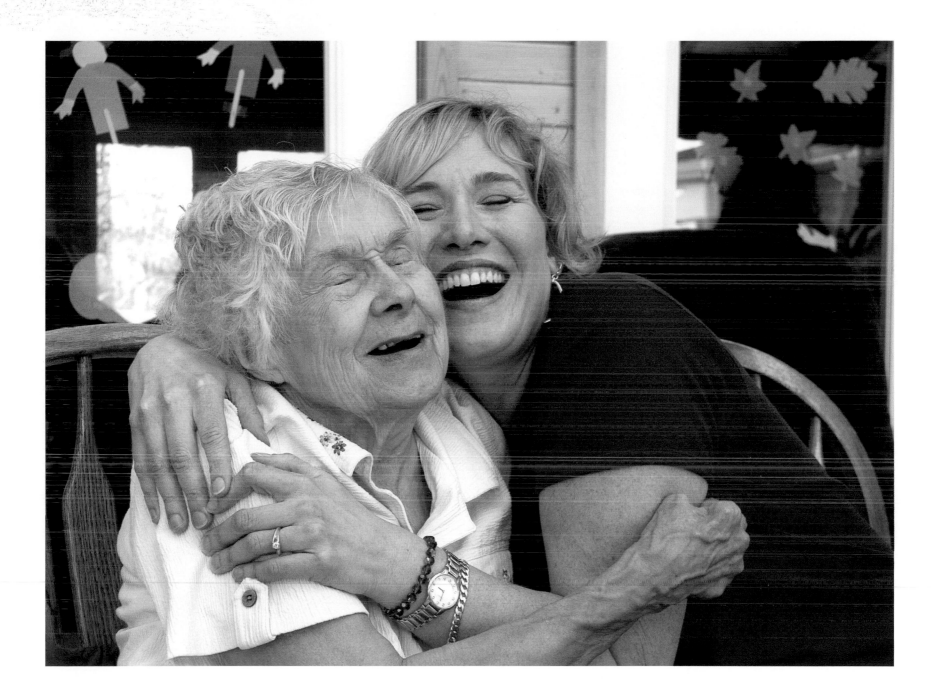

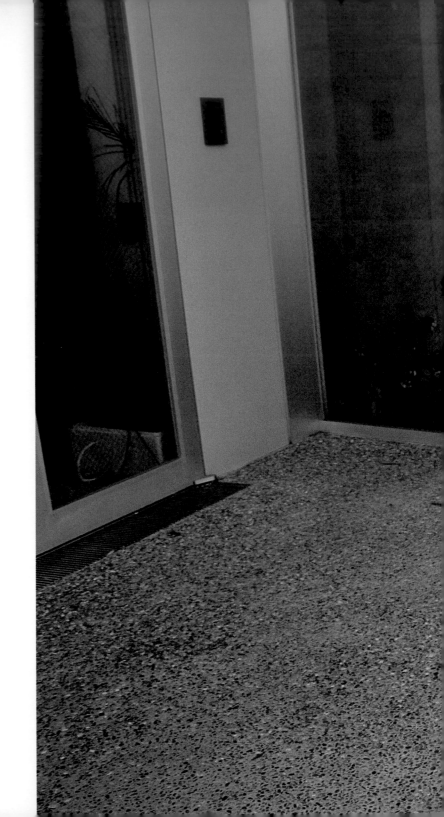

This luminous woman in gray is in harmony with the environment, and we witness a moment of peace. She seems to be so quiet, watching the bamboo. We can hear the sound of silence around her and inside her. Don't think that AD patients always need activities, group interactions, or anything special to do. Give them peaceful and beautiful places to live and rest. Allow them time for meditation or simply being in communication with life and nature.

—FRANÇOISE GUILLO-BEN AROUS, GERIATRICIAN

Enjoying the bamboo garden – Japan

The doors of this group home in suburban Kyoto are not locked, though there is careful supervision to ensure that residents do not leave the grounds unaccompanied. This woman loved going outdoors, breathing the fresh air, and admiring the bamboo garden next door. Quiet contemplation of nature is another way to celebrate life.

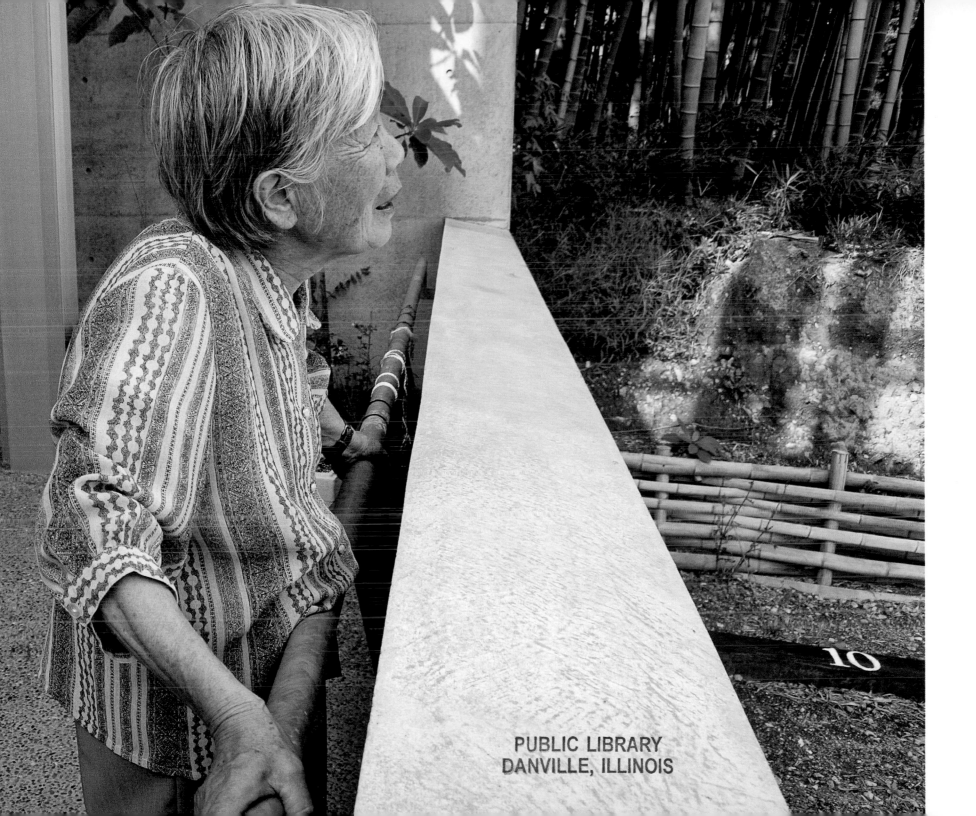

While making a documentary about Alzheimer's disease, and later a feature film about a family bonding through the challenges of memory loss, I came to see Alzheimer's as less of a disease and more of a canvas that helps us to explore the emotional tangles of care, affection, frustration, loss, void, irritation, guilt, and love. The canvas includes a range of poetic, lyrical, and practical problems, as the drama plays out on the islands of memory.

—BRAHMANAND S. SINGH, FILMMAKER

People diagnosed with Alzheimer's or a related dementia, as well as their families, often experience an overwhelming sense of hopelessness, mostly due to the symptoms and incurability of the disease. However, there's good news: There are proven techniques to successfully cope with this condition.

—KERRY MILLS, HEALTH-CARE PROFESSIONAL

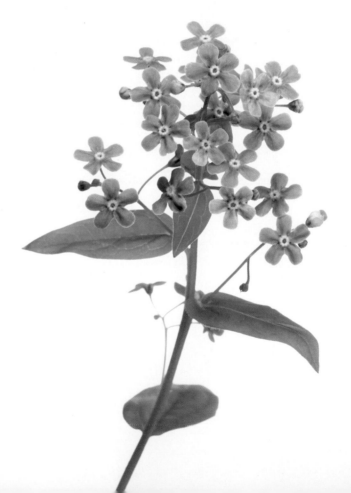

CHAPTER 3

CREATING PARTNERSHIPS

A family member—a husband or wife, a son or daughter, a brother or sister—usually becomes the primary caregiver to someone who develops a neurocognitive disorder. As the challenges to the person with dementia increase over the course of the illness, caregiving becomes increasingly difficult. There are many moving reports, oral and written, of great devotion and love. The presence of love, however, does not mean the absence of burden.

Assuring safety, meeting basic needs for food and hygiene, creating opportunities for social interaction, providing stimulation and affection, and simultaneously coping with aggressive behavior are particularly difficult when the caregiver lacks assistance from others. There is no substitute for the love of a family member, but caring strategies can be enhanced by learning how to better:

- understand the mechanisms of the illness
- adapt appropriate attitudes and behaviors toward the ill person
- communicate in order to maintain a relationship of exchange
- evaluate possibilities and know how to recognize limits

There is much to be gained by joining a permanent support group for exchange with others, conviviality, leisure, a chance to vent, conferences with presentations by experts, and more. These groups can also steer a caregiver to further outside assistance, trained and effective home-care aides, high-quality day programs, and professional counseling. Even with such partnerships, the burdens on family members are enormous. Without help, caregiver fatigue and poor health are common, and burnout is likely to occur. Numerous studies have shown that caregivers are prone to depression and high levels of stress. At some point a residential placement for the loved one may be desirable.

Support groups have also been created by and for people with early diagnosis. Members provide guidance and inspiration for maintaining morale and prolonging independence as well as tips for doing so. The Dementia Advocacy and Support Network (DASNI) online support group (www.dasninternational.org) gives information about groups in many languages.

Marcel Brasey, a dementia-care advocate, advises:

Become involved in your Alzheimer's associations. Join together with other diagnosed people, even beyond your borders. Thanks to the Internet, this has become possible. I myself realized that only those who live an identical situation can really fully understand. Between us, the communication is immediately easier. It is only through membership in a group of people with dementia, even if only virtual, that we can counteract the urge to become socially withdrawn and isolated.

In seeking a home-care aide, a day program, or a residential placement, caregivers are the key element. Neurologist Joan Amatniek reflects: "Who is the ideal caregiver? Someone who feels like the ideal granddaughter. She is the person who has the time to be with the AD person, to feel their presence, to react in a loving, individualized way. She is not the stressed person rushing to hand out pills, to ensure timely dressing or showering, or to stop wandering. Even when she is rushed to move on with her own life, she can make a moment of love feel like infinity."

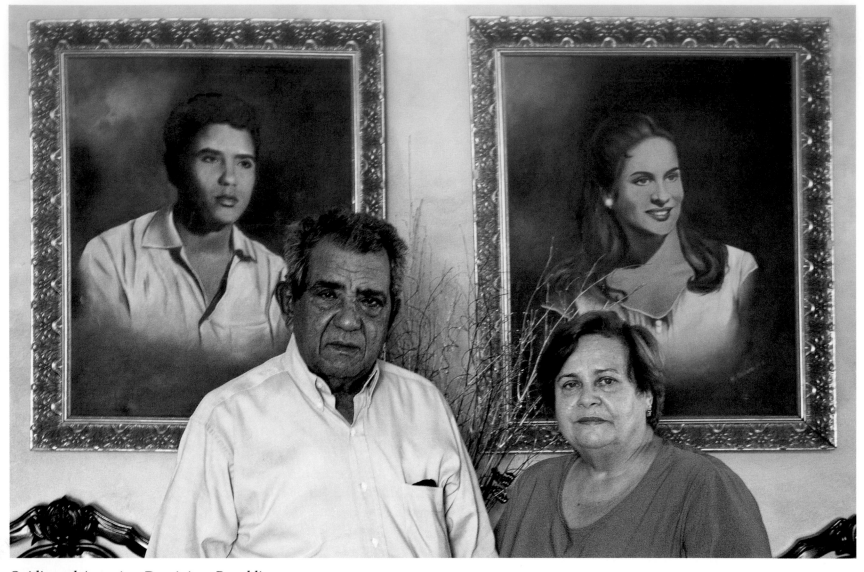

Ovidio and Antonia – Dominican Republic

Ovidio and Antonia have been married for fifty-one years. They stand before portraits made of them at ages twenty-nine and twenty-seven, now family treasures. They also treasure each other.

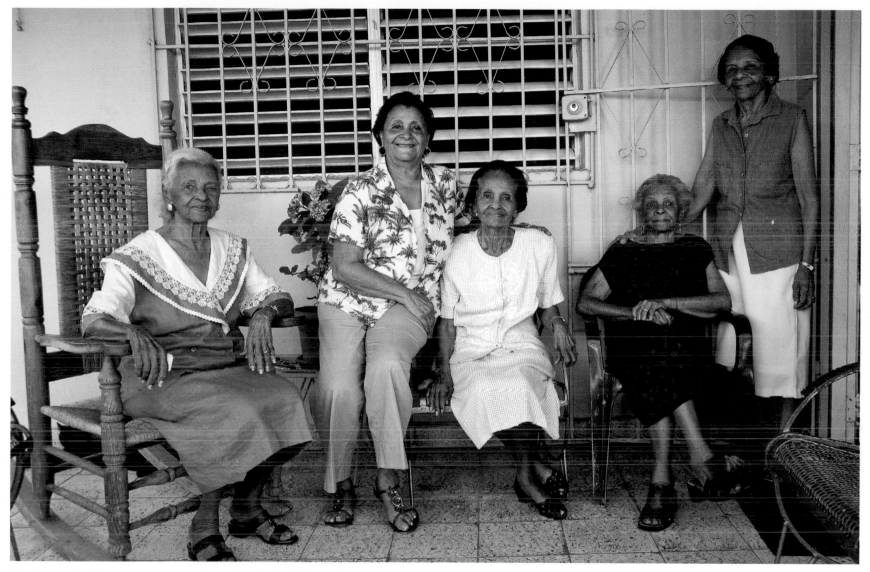

The Inocenio Lugo sisters at home – Dominican Republic

Altagracia Nuris (ninety-three), Arcelis (seventy-six), Mercedes (ninety-seven), Elsa (eighty-two), and Luz Candida (eighty) live in the same house and help one another with all aspects of life. One of their key responsibilities is caring for Elsa as her Alzheimer's advances.

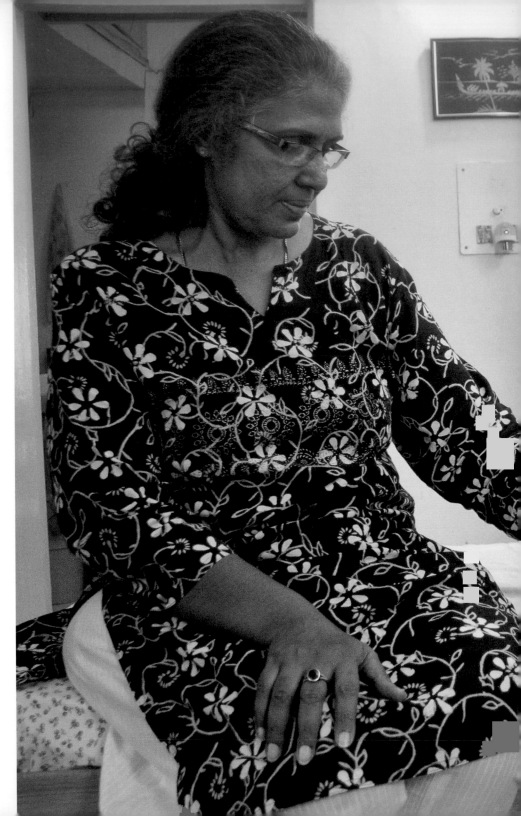

The tragedy of Alzheimer's disease is in its potential to destroy relationships. It is understandable why spouses, adult children, other relatives, and friends feel such terrible grief. What is hopeful is that so many loved ones move beyond their denial, anger, and sadness to some measure of acceptance. They learn to reconfigure the relationship, let go of the past, and live in the here and now. These stories need to be told, too, in order to bear witness to courage in the face of adversity. Alzheimer's disease does not have to end a relationship but will indeed radically change it.

—DANIEL KUHN, COMMUNITY EDUCATOR

Deepika, caregiver for her father – India

Deepika was working as a successful human rights activist when her father was diagnosed with Alzheimer's disease. She soon found herself his full-time caregiver, and she shifted to working from home. As his condition worsened, she was forced to cut back on the time she spent on her career. This meant reduced income. Deepika's devotion was strong, but when I met her she was exhausted and seemed to be suffering from caregiver burnout. Up to that point, she'd had no assistance in caregiving for seven years; the Alzheimer's and Related Disorders Society of India (ARDSI) had just helped her find an aide.

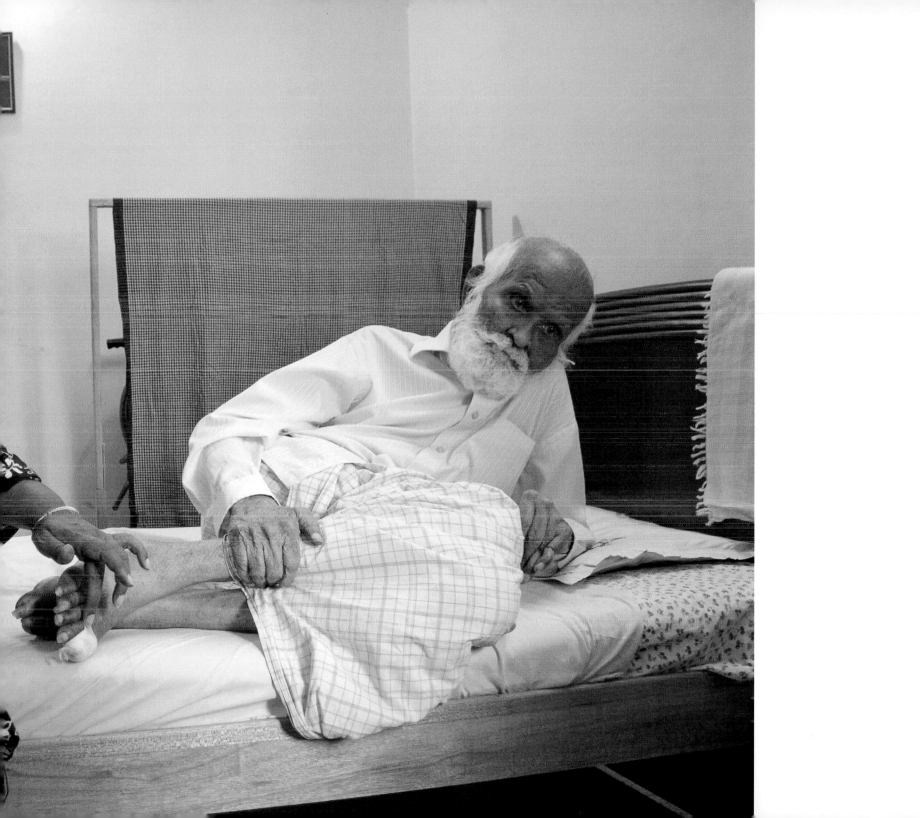

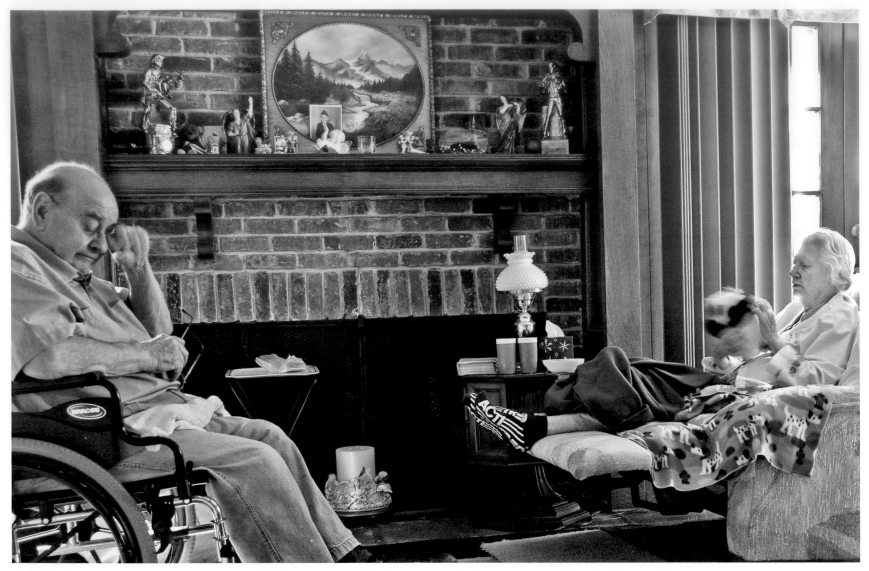

Houston couple in their living room – USA

Joe chose to care for his wife, Luleene, at home, with assistance from a home-care facility and more recently, from hospice. Luleene was a musician who played the organ and sang, so a music therapist visit was included in the weekly program designed for her. More than one hundred china and glass figurines of dogs decorate rooms in their Texas home, and visits from real dogs in a pet therapy program are special treats. Like many other devoted caregivers, Joe has paid less attention to his own medical needs while focusing on Luleene's needs during several years of end-stage dementia.

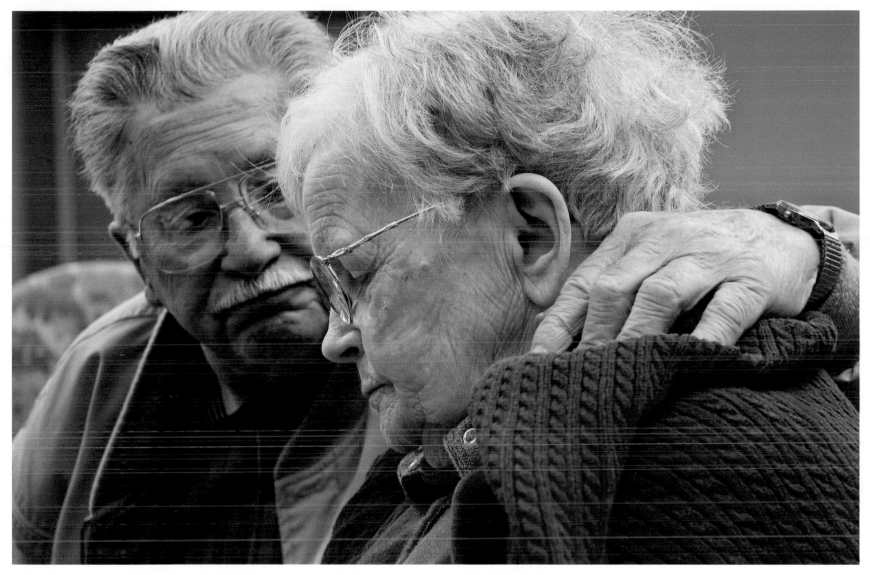

"I'd give you my Bronze Star if you could bring her back"–USA

Len and Bette have been married for sixty-three years. He cared for her at home in the first years of her cognitive difficulties, until wandering and other problems led both the doctor and their children to urge an institutional placement. Len is consumed by her losses and his own. He told me, "I've left everything in the house the way it used to be as if she might come home. But in the long run, I know it's not true. I've lost her. She's here but I've lost her. I'd give you my Bronze Star if you could bring her back."

The availability of help for family members varies from country to country and from community to community within the same smaller geographic area.

Traditionally in Asia, older people have been respected and taken care of by family members. Family norms have changed drastically due to unprecedented demographic transition, landing us in a hitherto unthinkable era of longevity and creating an urgent need to develop new programs of care for the elderly. For the primary caregiver of a person with dementia, real respite would mean a short vacation or, in its simplest form, a home aide or a trained caregiver who works a several-hour shift. In India, moving the person to a facility is not at all common.

One of the biggest challenges lies in the provision of adequate and accessible day services for dementia patients. These are being developed, but more are needed. Even when several options are available, family members need help in exploring ideas of how to best use them. The strain on family members who don't get a break is reflected in higher rates of depression, hypertension, diabetes, sleep disorder, heart disease, and death. We need to assist them in finding ways to care for themselves while caring for a loved one.

—NIRMALA NARULA, ALZHEIMER'S ADVOCATE

Vijay was a chief executive in one of India's top companies. Ten years ago, when he was fifty-two, he and his wife, Anu, were told that his increasing problems were due to early-onset Alzheimer's. They were not prepared for this news, but Anu managed the family life and become the sole earner. She pursued many avenues to find what Vijay needed: a day-care center, a home caregiver, homeopathic medicine. Anu also sought out and benefited from advice and assistance from others, and she joined a support group. She and her family members learned meditation to deal with stress. She loves Vijay very much and benefits from the assistance of Mr. Deepak, the caregiver seen here feeding Vijay.

Anu now offers support and advice to other caregivers through ARDSI, and she willingly shares her story through the mass media to create better understanding and fight stigma.

—SAILESH MISHRA, HEALTH PROFESSIONAL

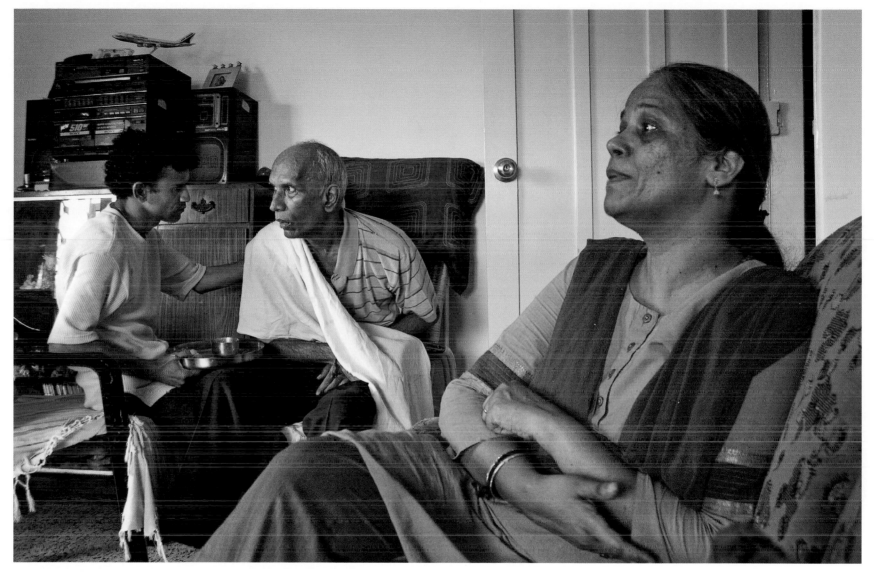

Anu with her husband, Vijay, and an aide – India

Anu has been courageous and effective in caring for her husband. She sought and found assistance in the form of advice, and later an aide. Now she helps others do the same.

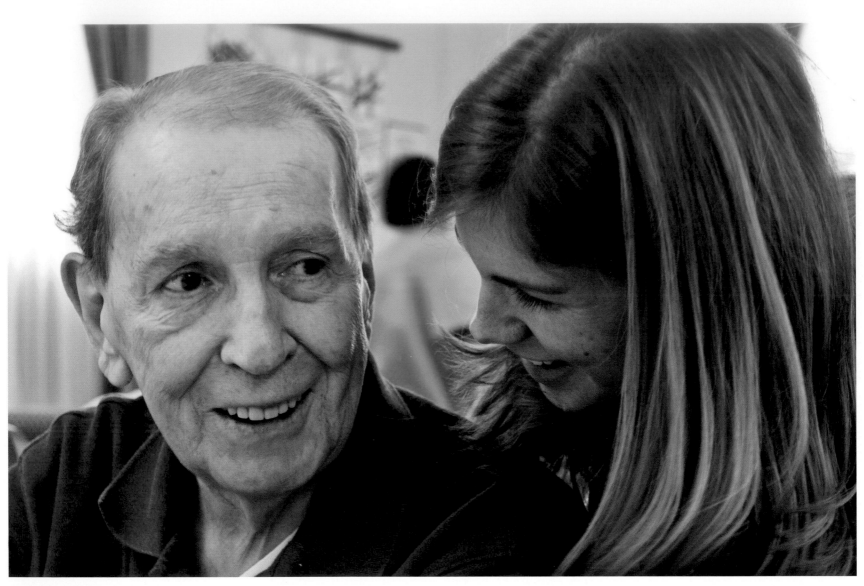

Kerry makes Tunc and everyone else smile – USA

Caregiver Kerry Mills brings sunshine into the room with her presence, and every resident seems to respond to her. Kerry knows how to "put it all together"—to relate to patients, family, and staff. She quickly moved from being an activity director, to the director of a residential community, to a regional coordinator. Now she serves as an independent "dementia coach" through her company, Engaging Alzheimer's.

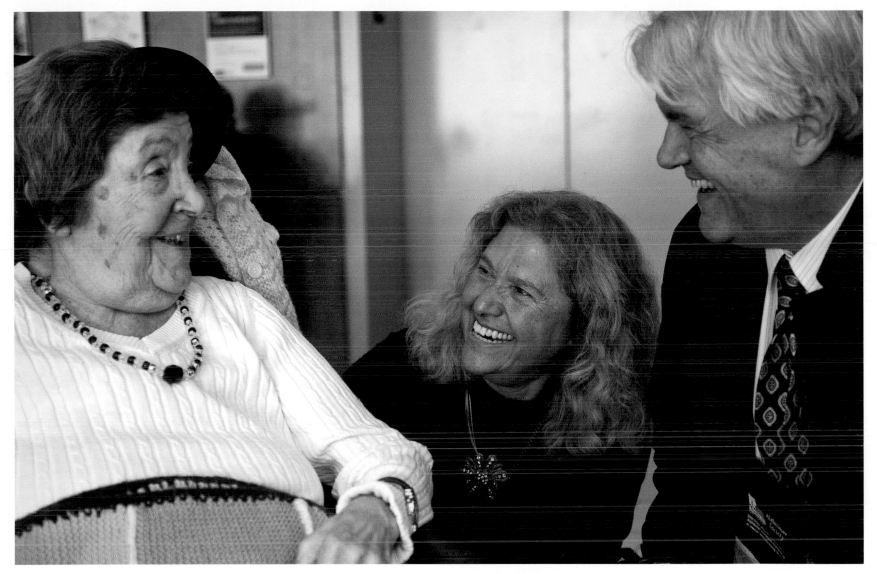

Anna with her daughter, Louanna, and Dr. Peter Whitehouse – Canada

Anna led an extraordinarily rich life, working from her teens until her late seventies, then part-time until her mid-eighties, all while raising two children. She was also active in local politics, and volunteered in a number of community organizations up to her diagnosis with moderate dementia a few days before her ninety-fourth birthday. Now at ninety-seven, she has taken up drumming and tai chi at the facility where she resides. She loves family visits and meeting new people.

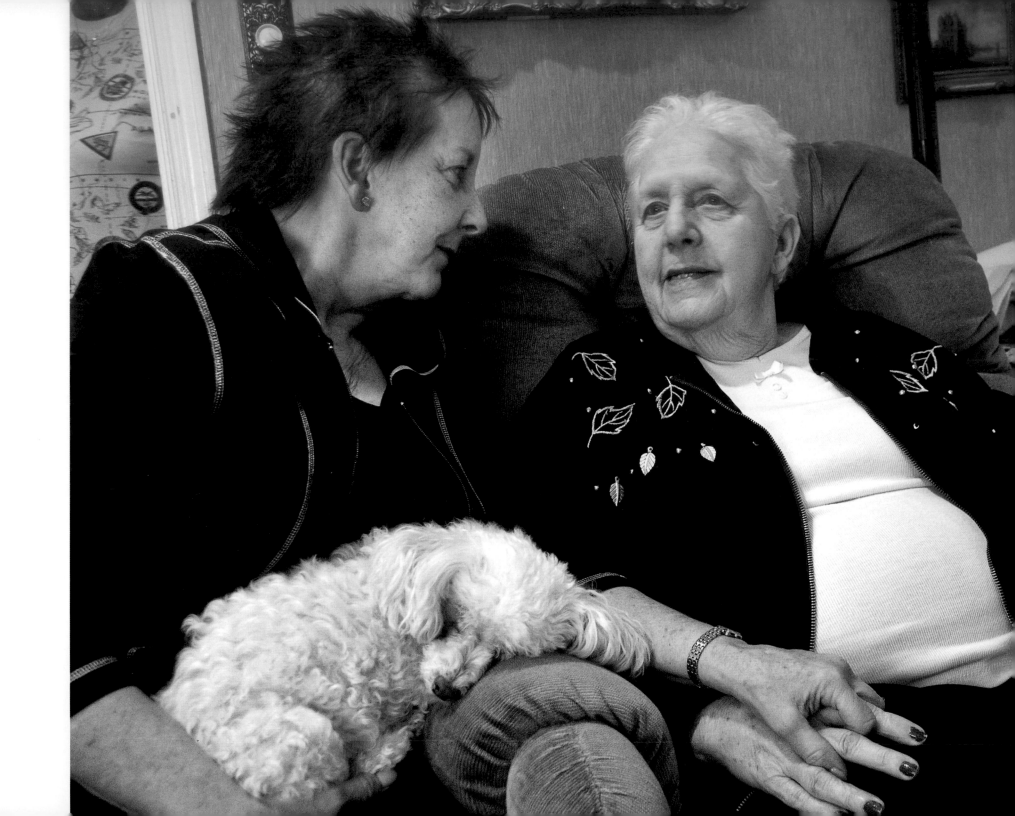

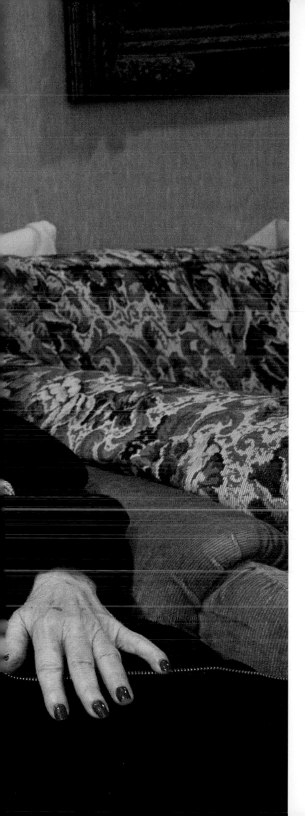

This photograph makes me think of a comment by Colette Roumanoff, a French theater director whose husband was diagnosed with Alzheimer's disease. She said, "In illness, for me it is very important to distinguish among memory, intelligence, and sensitivity. These are three different domains. Illness does not alter intelligence or sensibility. On the contrary, sensitivity increases."

—ANNE-CLAUDE JUILLERAT, PSYCHOLOGIST

Helen Jr. and Helen Sr. holding hands – USA

Helen Sr. has been experiencing moderate dementia for the past ten years. She was a prolific artist through the early stages of her dementia, until she lost her eyesight. Her oil paintings adorn the walls of Helen Jr.'s home as well as those of many family members, friends, and those who purchased her artwork from the 1960s through the 1980s. For the past three years, Helen Sr. has been living at a small, private, residential group home near Washington, DC, for people with dementia. Her daughter, Helen Jr., and other family members live in the area and visit regularly. They feel that here every person, from residents to family members and caregivers, is family.

Bob DeMarco's daily blogs at www.alzheimersreadingroom.com provide insights and ideas for everyone. In this abbreviated post, he offers ideas about how you can help as a friend of an Alzheimer's caregiver. You can make a big difference!

HOW FRIENDS CAN HELP CAREGIVERS

One issue that really frustrates me is the treatment of Alzheimer's caregivers. Most hear people tell them how wonderful they are for taking care of their loved one. As a caregiver, I learned to appreciate these compliments. They help, they really do. However, if you have a loved one, family member, or friend who is an Alzheimer's caregiver and all you do is tell them what a great job they are doing—it is not enough. Many Alzheimer's caregivers are forgotten by family and friends. This is a sad truth that is rarely discussed.

I meet and talk to caregivers all the time. It is not unusual for them to tell me that as time goes on, and as Alzheimer's worsens, one by one their family and friends fade away. This is understandable—Alzheimer's is scary and disconcerting. It is hard to accept, hard to understand, and hard to watch as it progresses.

It is not unusual for the friends and family to continue to call and give the caregiver the old "rah rah siss boom ba" and then get back to their own lives. Meanwhile, the caregiver puts her or his life on hold—or worse, has no life—while caring for an Alzheimer's sufferer. Calling and letting the caregiver vent is helpful, very helpful, but it is not enough.

Like it or not, if you are a family member or friend of an Alzheimer's caregiver and you are not helping them, you have abandoned them. I am sure this sounds harsh. But it's not even close to the harshness of your own behavior.

Caregivers need help. A few hours here and there to get away from it all is an important step in improving their lives. Give them some time to enjoy the world outside their home—time to reconnect with others.

Why am I so passionate and adamant about this?

Forty percent of Alzheimer's caregivers end up suffering from depression: four out of ten. Do you want to see this happen to a loved one or friend? Alzheimer's is a sinister disease—it kills the brain of the person suffering from Alzheimer's. And it will try to kill the brain of the Alzheimer's caregiver. I really don't believe this problem is well understood.

Here are my immediate suggestions:

- *If you know an Alzheimer's caregiver, find a way to organize the troops—family and friends—and get involved. Somebody has to take the initiative, and if you are reading this, take charge now. Nothing works better than a small team of caregiver-helpers. The key words here are team and teamwork.*

- *Alzheimer's caregivers need to get away from it all. They need a respite every few days. This means someone must take over while they go do something they enjoy. You might find this difficult to believe, but when I get the chance to go to the store, take my time, and look around at the surroundings—it is a treat. I bet you take this for granted.*
- *Invite your Alzheimer's caregiver and their loved one over for lunch or dinner. Most Alzheimer's caregivers tell me that one of the biggest problems they face is socialization. If you don't believe me, ask them. Both the caregiver and patient need to talk and interact with other human beings. Don't you? Socializing really benefits the Alzheimer's sufferer. What is not as apparent is how much it benefits the Alzheimer's caregiver.*
- *Many sufferers of Alzheimer's get up in the middle of the night. This means the caregiver needs to get up with them. Sleep deprivation often leads to depression, and it can cause erratic behavior. Imagine going night after night without sleeping well. If this is happening to someone you know, you need to help design a plan that allows them to get the sleep they need.*
- *Do you know an Alzheimer's caregiver? Ask them the last time they went out to see a movie. You might be surprised when you hear the answer. You can solve this problem through teamwork: One person looks after the patient, and the other takes the caregiver to the movie. This is a "get away from it all experience" that is really beneficial to the mental health of the Alzheimer's caregiver.*

I know from my own experience that if you take action, you'll end up feeling good about yourself. Action will change and enrich your life. Don't allow Alzheimer's to take control of the caregiver—form a team to take control of the problem. The caregiver gets a life, the sufferer gets more effective care, and the team gets the wonderful feeling that comes from doing something and getting involved.

—BOB DEMARCO, FOUNDER/EDITOR, THE ALZHEIMER'S READING ROOM

WHEN A RESIDENTIAL PLACEMENT IS DESIRED

I believe that placing someone with Alzheimer's in a residential facility should not be thought of as a last resort when all else fails. Teams of loving, trained personnel with a person-centered approach can provide more energy and stimulation than can a family caregiver. When they become partners with a facility, family members can focus on what they can do best. The photos in this book show many stellar programs, but as of now there are not enough of them. Places that provide "warehousing," unimaginative programming, and overuse of psychotropic medications are more common. It is important to do research.

Louanna Cocchiarella (see page 41) didn't need to do much research when her mother, Anna, required more assistance. Anna had been an active volunteer at Baycrest for more than fifty-five years, working in the abilities store, the creative arts center, the cafeteria, the hospital, at events, and in the home for the aged. Following her diagnosis with moderate dementia, she began attending the Baycrest Day Center Program.

A year and a half later, at age ninety-five, Anna moved into Baycrest's Apotex residential center. Louanna reports:

Anna herself chose to make the move, feeling it was not a move out of her community and into a nursing home, but rather a move to the heart of her lifelong community. My mother's life is far better than it could possibly be if she stayed "at home." Baycrest is a vibrant and loving place where my mother receives wonderful care and has opportunities that make her life rich with experiences, meaning, learning, and growth.

Most people have neither the knowledge of nor respect for a nearby institution, nor the foresight or courage to put their names on a waiting list, which often must be done long before the time they need a placement. Laura Bramly's experience was quite negative. It has led her to actively blogging, writing, and working as an Alzheimer's advocate to enlighten and advise others:

I am often asked what I would do differently for my mother, knowing what I know now. In June 2009 at the age of eighty-seven, my mother passed away from vascular dementia. For sure, if I could do it again, I would seek the wonderful and sophisticated level of memory care that is available in facilities such as those shown in this book. I would have done everything I could to get her into one.

My mother was "promoted" to the locked dementia-care unit at her long-term-care home because of her behavior. She was not violent or angry, but she called out many, many times during the day and night for her husband, as he was the only person she recognized and trusted. Because the staff didn't have time to constantly answer her calls for help or John, and because her calling out was disturbing to other residents, she was moved to dementia care. This move contributed to her rapid decline, but we didn't know that better dementia care was available, or what even constituted better care. We didn't know what we were looking for or that we should be looking for it in the first place. Now I do.

Hope and work for the best; prepare for the worst. A placement in a high-quality community can provide a positive environment for Alzheimer's patients and loved ones alike.

HOW TO CHOOSE A NURSING HOME FOR YOUR LOVED ONE WITH ALZHEIMER'S OR OTHER DEMENTIAS

A recent study found that seniors' greatest fears are the loss of independence (26 percent), and being forced to move out of their homes and into a nursing facility (13 percent). By contrast, only 3 percent most fear dying or death. Transitioning your senior into a nursing home is certainly one of the hardest decisions you'll make. But when your loved one is an Alzheimer's or dementia sufferer, or someone who requires post-incident (such as stroke or broken hip) rehabilitation, fully 60 percent of these decisions are made by hospitals. The unfortunate reality is that the hospital needs an early discharge; it's motivated to find an available nursing home bed, whatever the operator's quality or reputation. Under these circumstances, you'll have to intervene quickly, and you might not have sufficient information to make a good decision about the nursing home placement. Fortunately, there are abundant helpful resources. Here are a few suggestions:

Get the facts. The Centers for Medicare and Medicaid Services collect data for the nation's nursing homes (on topics such as health inspections, staffing, and quality measures) and produce a one- to five-star rating. You can view this online at www.medicare.gov/nhcompare. Click on Find and Compare Nursing Homes to search for nursing homes by name, zip code, city, state, and county. Also on this website, a box invites you to click for additional information about the rating system itself. and you'll find an informative, downloadable brochure on the site (http://tinyurl.com/3ntd5wt) titled *Guide to Choosing a Nursing Home.*

Make a personal visit. As useful as background information is, there's no substitute for making a visit—or several—to prospective nursing homes. Take along the checklist from the Nursing Home Compare site (www.medicare.gov/nursing/checklist.pdf). During your visit, use your five senses, and trust them! What does the place smell like? Are staff members friendly? How do they interact with the residents? And perhaps most important: Is the facility alive with activity or are some—or many—of the residents strapped into their wheelchairs, listless and unresponsive? If so, what you're probably witnessing is not a side effect of dementia, but rather the all-too-common practice of overmedicating residents as a substitute for personal care.

Ask questions. Meet the director of the facility, the lead physician, and the head nurse. You'll want to know whether they practice person-centered care. Most nursing homes are run like military boot camps—residents are required to wake up, have meals, bathe, and go to bed at the same times. Conversely, person-centered care encourages residents to set up their own individualized schedules for these activities. Inquire about staff turnover and whether you may attend a resident council meeting. High annual turnover—above 30 percent—is typical. The resident council is an opportunity for residents and their families to discuss problems and offer ideas for improvements.

Seek other resources. Every state has a federally funded long-term-care ombudsman who advocates on behalf of nursing home residents. This person may have useful information about particular nursing homes that supplements the Medicare ratings, including health inspection reports and complaints, both of which are public information. You can find the one in your area via www.ltcombudsman.org/ombudsman.

—LAURENCE HARMON, LAWYER

I conduct training programs with professionals who care for people with dementia. I remind them that one of the simplest acts of love is to look people in their eyes, call them by their preferred name, and offer a smile, a handshake, and a warm greeting or compliment. Imagine if this brief interaction was repeated many times per day by everyone who worked there: Identity would be preserved, self-esteem would be elevated, and human bonds would be strengthened.

—DANIEL KUHN, COMMUNITY EDUCATOR

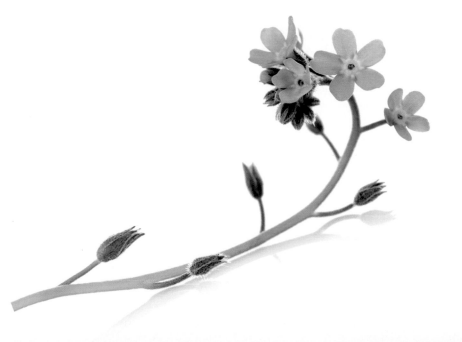

CHAPTER 4

INCREASING CONFIDENCE AND CONNECTION

Alzheimer's and related disorders interrupt and confound the lives of those who are directly affected and those who provide care. Physical symptoms increase in severity over time, creating progressively greater challenges to patients and caretakers. Reduced self-confidence is among the most common results of not only a deteriorating medical condition, but also shifting social factors: loss of employment, loss of abilities and activities, and loss of independence. A major task for family, friends, volunteers, and residential or day-care staff is to help the person with dementia reinvigorate self-confidence.

Those who employ a person-centered approach have developed effective ways to reduce isolation, relieve fear, and bring pleasure. They address the people they care for with respect and make emotional connections with each, validating the person as a person. These connections play a major role in determining whether someone withers or flourishes. Recipients of validation, affection, and enjoyment often pass it on to others. They also laugh more. This is in marked contrast with the use of antipsychotics to deal with aggressive behavior.

Children and animals can also play a role in increasing confidence and connection. When grandchildren or other young family members are present, the atmosphere feels more like "real life." Young people generally engage in playful, open communication more easily than most adults. Excellent programs have been successful in linking children and adolescents to older people with dementia who are not their relatives.

Animals create a sense of emotional safety for many people. They may also open channels of nonthreatening communication among a person with dementia and family members, care professionals, and other participants in a day or residential program. Whether the animal is a personal pet, a pet therapy visitor, or a resident of the community, its presence can create a brighter atmosphere and a stronger sense of connection.

Changing the culture of care for people with dementia involves attention to their environmental and architectural surroundings as well as to the social and psychological challenges. Researchers have offered fascinating assessments and practical advice concerning the interactions among visual impairments, cognitive challenges, and architecture. John Zeisel lists eight physical environment elements that correlate with reduction of symptoms: exit control, walking paths, privacy, shared spaces, gardens, home-like quality, sensory understanding, and supports for independence and empowerment.

Books by Margaret Calkins, John Zeisel, and Joanne Koenig Coste (see the resources section) include guidelines for adjusting home and professional spaces. They recommend many simple physical changes that can help reduce stress, increase sociability, diminish confusion, and provide a stronger predictability in personal territory.

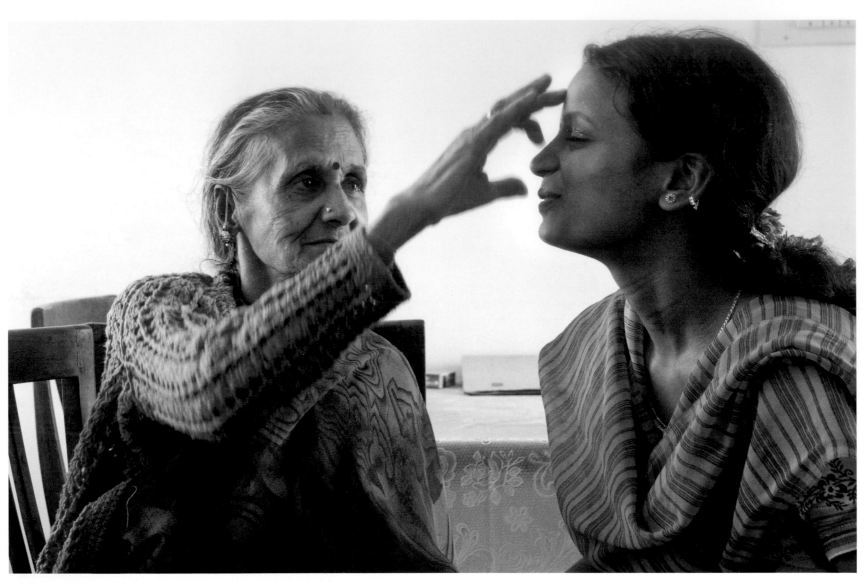

Bhanumathi brushing away the evil spirits from an aide – India

Bhanumathi frequently performs a finger ritual to ward off evil spirits and also to show that she is caring and loving to all the aides at the Nightingales day program in Bangalore, India.

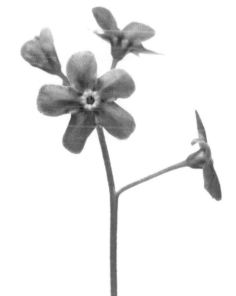

WHAT CARE DO WE WANT TO SEE FOR PEOPLE WITH DEMENTIA?

Care that upholds both their and our sense of humanity, sense of goodness, sense of giving . . .

- *compassion for the person*
- *contact with the person*
- *involving the person*
- *celebrating the person*
- *being with the person*
- *reminding the person who she is*
- *holding the person's pain and sharing his joy*
- *being with the person in her silence*
- *reaching to where the person is*
- *letting the person be separate and alone*
- *accepting the person's gifts*
- *guiding the person to what he can do*
- *seeing the light in the person's eyes*
- *looking the person in the eye*
- *bringing the person into the world*
- *shielding the person from the world*
- *giving the person affection*
- *giving the person time*
- *honoring the living person*

—MURNA DOWNS, PROFESSOR OF DEMENTIA STUDIES

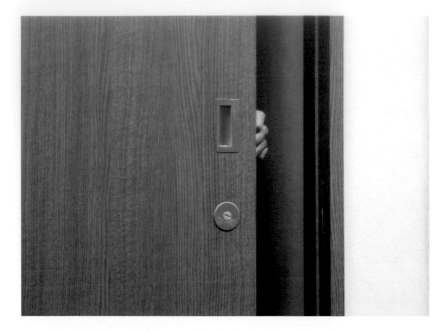

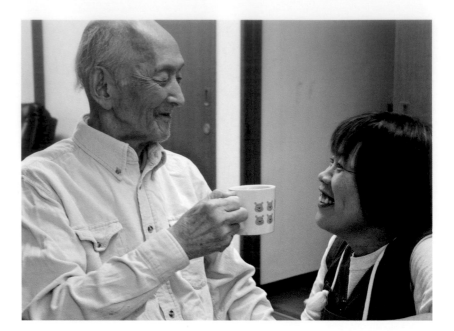

Helping the shy man – Japan

This resident of a Kyoto group home was often fearful about leaving his room to interact with the other eight residents. The excellent staff, however, knew how to bring him to safely engage with others. Here an aide entices him into the common area and makes him comfortable with tea, smiles, and a soft voice. Next the director plays music from the man's youth and invites him to dance. Then he sits in the sunlight with another resident, Mrs. Morimoto, and they converse for more than fifteen minutes, though neither is any longer able to speak in full sentences.

Giving witness to others, participating with them, are the bases of clinical research.

—PHILIPPE ROBERT, PSYCHIATRIST

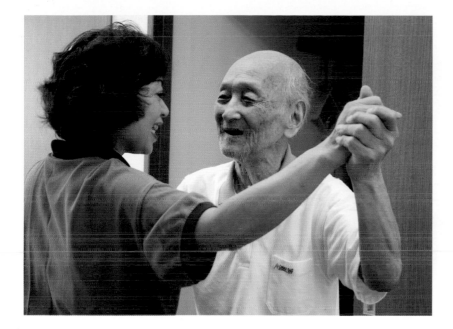

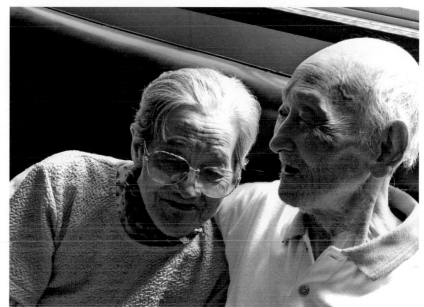

I once met two women with advanced Alzheimer's disease who had become best friends while living in a nursing home. But their friendship defied the usual definition because they did not share the same language. One woman spoke English but her words and grammar were severely impaired. The other woman had known English but reverted mainly to her native Japanese. How they communicated was unclear to the casual observer. Words alone meant little, if anything, to them. They had moved beyond language. It was something to behold.

—DANIEL KUHN, COMMUNITY EDUCATOR

There are many ways photographs can dramatically change the image people suffering from a fatal illness develop about themselves. Taking a photo means considering the patient as a person, and looking at him or her with a complete availability, curiosity, human and artistic sensitivity. If you make a portrait "in majesty," or any photograph that represents a special moment, you will learn and share a great deal about the subject's past and present thoughts, fears, or pride. Both self-esteem and self-image are enhanced and reinforced. In your picture, they are no longer Alzheimer's patients but perhaps former war heroes or outstanding mothers who can think and say, "Hey, look—that's me!"

Communicating through a photograph deeply influences the relationship between the family members and the patient, and between the medical team and the patient.

—FRANÇOISE GUILLO-BEN AROUS, GERIATRICIAN

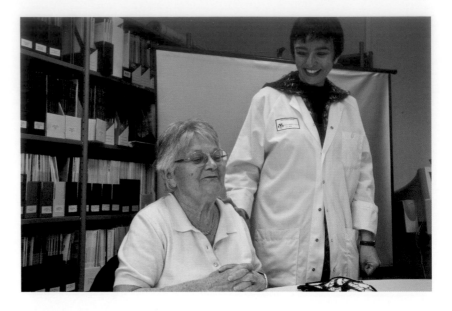

Marie Antoinette, pleased to have remembered – France
A well-run memory clinic can provide more than the strengthening of cognitive skills. Encouragement and praise can lift self-esteem. Marie Antoinette appreciated the patience and reinforcement of her efforts by Christelle, the clinic psychologist running the session.

Françoise Guillo at the CMRR photo gallery – France
The Alzheimer's service in Nice, initially divided between two buildings, was joined a few years ago by a long, empty basement corridor. Professor Robert, worried that the participants in the memory clinic would feel devalued by this unattractive space, asked me to take their portraits during their sessions, which he then used to line the walls of the hall. When the thirty-two large prints were put up, participants were excited and felt it was "their" place.

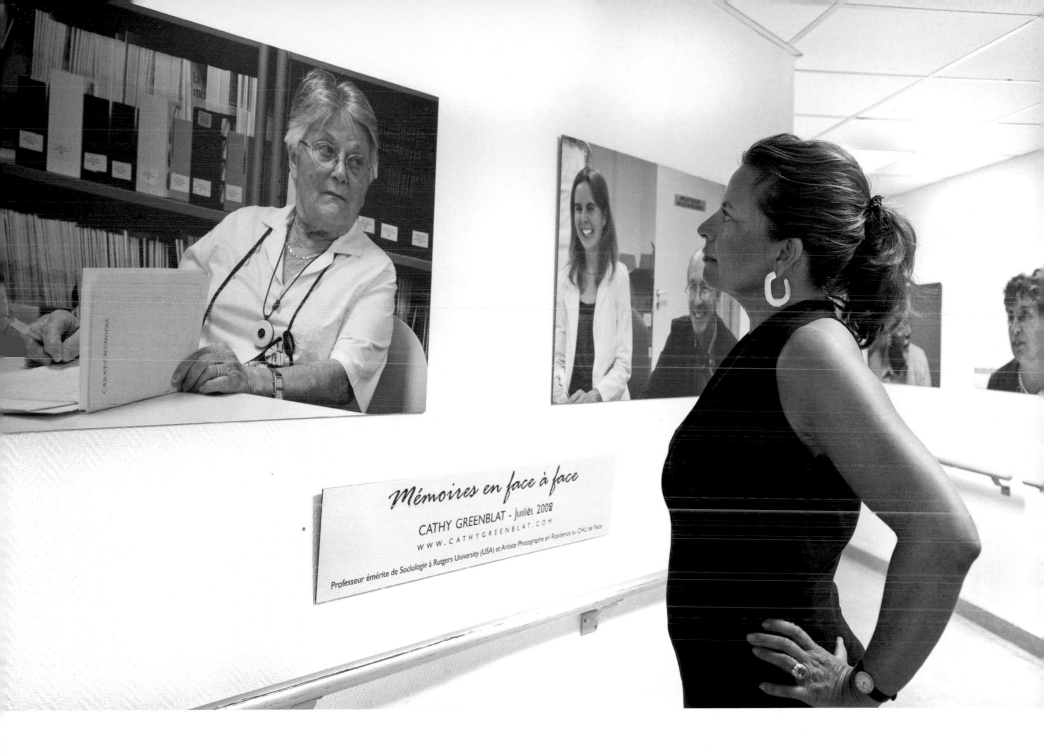

Mémoires en face à face

CATHY GREENBLAT - Juillet 2008

WWW.CATHYGREENBLAT.COM

Professeur émérite de Sociologie à Rutgers University (USA) et Artiste Photographe en Résidence au CHU de Nice

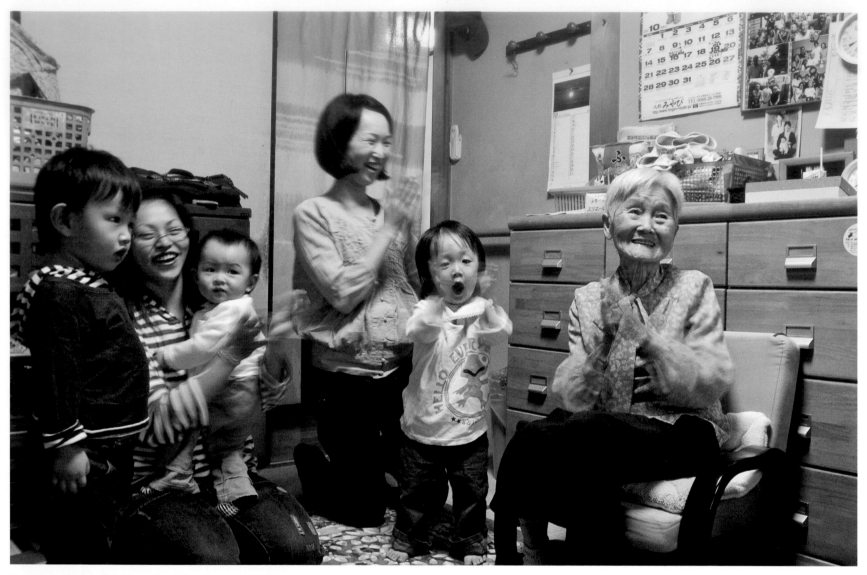

Family singing "Happy Birthday" to Mrs. Hamajma, eighty-eight – Japan

On Mrs. Hamajma's eighty-eighth birthday, neither her husband's terminal illness nor her advanced Alzheimer's disease prevented her from enjoying the time with her family, who sang "Happy Birthday" with exuberance.

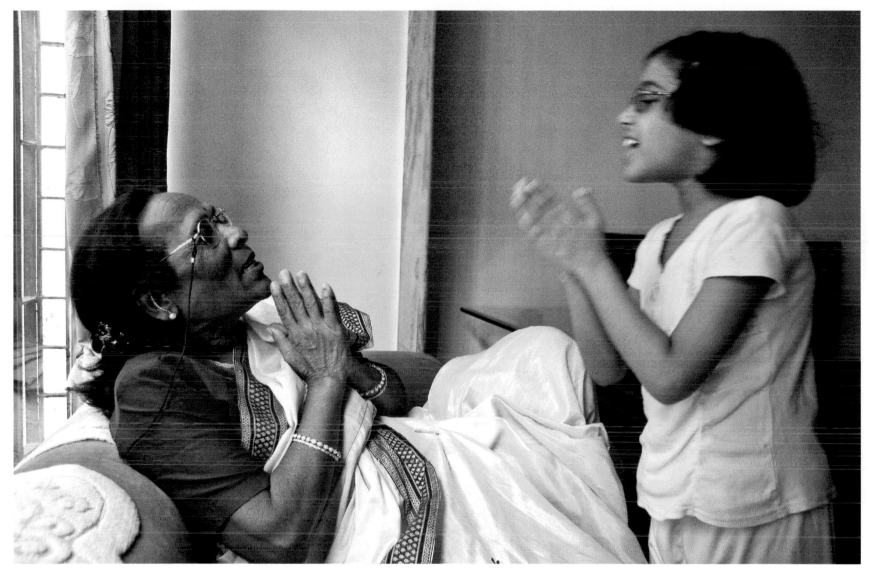

Srushti chanting with her grandmother   India

As Mandakini became increasingly confused, she found she could no longer live alone. Two of her sons were fearful of taking her in because they had young children. Her third son, Satish, and his wife, Neha, brought her to their home, where they engaged the assistance of a professional caregiver.

Here eight-year old Srushti leads her grandmother in the religious chants that have been important to her throughout her life. Srushti is proud to have an important role in the family.

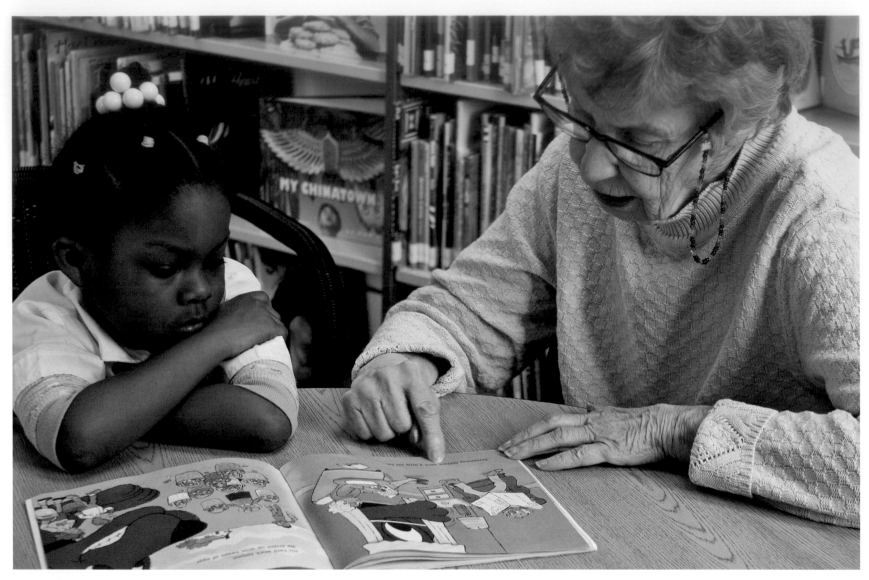

Erin and Jean at The Intergenerational School – USA

Jean was part of a team of volunteers who regularly came to The Intergenerational School in Cleveland, Ohio. She spent several hours this day in the library, helping students improve their reading skills.

Two projects that have greatly impressed me are The Intergenerational School (TIS) in Cleveland and the Memory Bridge Project based in Chicago.

TIS is a public charter school created in 2000 by Drs. Cathy and Peter Whitehouse. It embodies two mainstay principles:

1. Learning is a lifelong developmental process.
2. Knowledge is socially constructed.

One of the school's many innovative elements is the regular presence of seniors and other community members, including several with age-associated cognitive challenges ranging from mild to relatively severe. They share time and wisdom with TIS students through a number of intergenerational learning programs: as reading mentors or computer/art museum explorers, and through gardening, narrative histories, and senior home partners.

Dr. Cathy Whitehouse reports that an important moment for the school came with her realization that even someone with dementia could still read a children's book. "When Barbara is sitting with a child and reading, she's able to interact with the child in the moment. I firmly believe that she enjoys the time she spends here, and if she doesn't remember it five minutes later, it doesn't matter. It's just been great to have her."

At a recent "volunteer of the year" award ceremony, the recipient asked her daughter why she was receiving this recognition. Her daughter reminded her that she came to the school every week to read to the kids, and that they loved it. Although the awardee did not retain these short-term memories, she was assured that the children remembered just how helpful she was.

The Memory Bridge Initiative is dedicated to keeping people with dementia meaningfully connected to others. Their flagship program is a twelve-week after-school program funded by the Illinois Department of Human Services. Junior and senior high school students are educated about Alzheimer's disease and related issues and then paired with a person living with Alzheimer's.

The two meet four times and exchange letters. Founder/president Michael Verde reports that the program benefits students in many ways, including helping them to develop their emotional and social intelligence. Participants from long-term-care facilities are helped to feel more connected to people in their community.

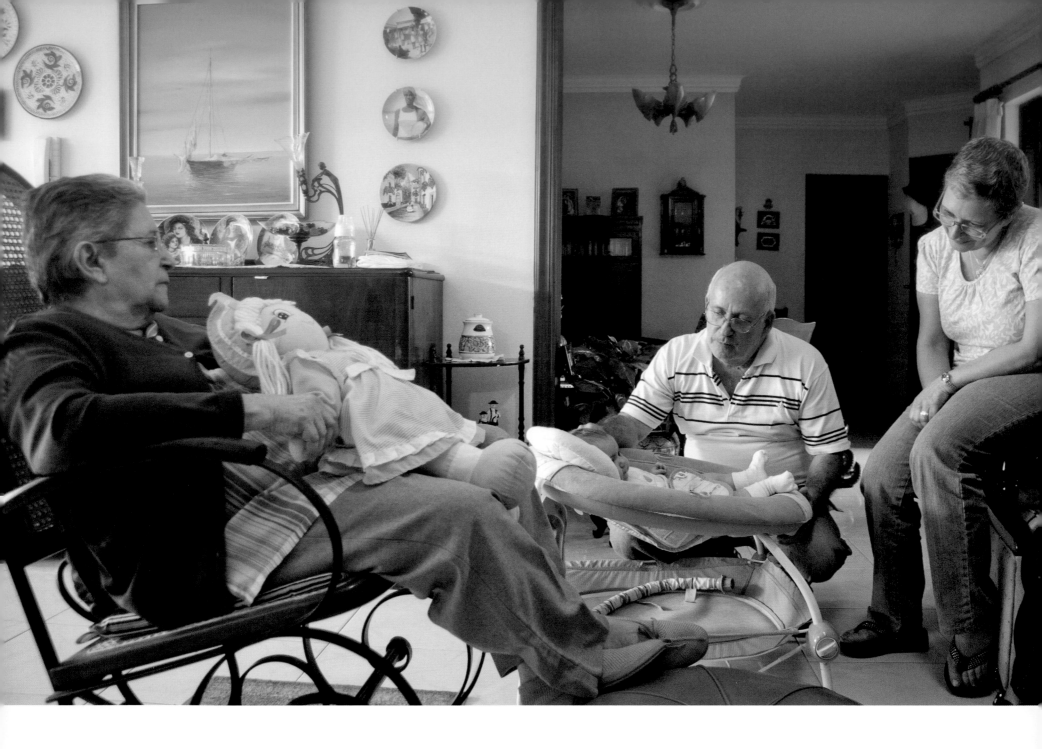

Dolls can be very useful in comforting some patients. I had a patient who used to scream constantly—the whole neighborhood could hear her. Dolls turned out to be the solution. She spent the whole day washing three dolls, combing their hair, changing their clothes, et cetera. She felt useful again and that she had a job to do. Another patient of mine was a doctor who wandered around his big house aimlessly and anxiously, as if he had something he had to do. I learned that he wanted to go to the hospital to see his patients, as one "was very ill and dying." He began to confuse his wife with a patient. He didn't want her to move as "she was just operated on." Because the house was big with many rooms, we acquired some dummies (used by the Red Cross to teach) and put them in the beds in three rooms. He loved that. He spent the whole day entering each of those rooms, "examining" each patient, and asking everybody to be quiet as the patients were resting. His wife was sad to see her husband doing this, but she was also relieved and he was much calmer.

—DAISY ACOSTA, PSYCHIATRIST

Olga, Carlos, Flerida, a doll, and a great-grandchild – Dominican Republic

Olga, eighty-nine, now lives with one of her daughters, Flerida, and Flerida's husband, Carlos. They often have visits from their children and grandchildren. As they attend to Olga's youngest great-grandchild, Olga holds a doll that helps to keep her calm.

Pet therapy programs such as Silverado Hospice's Silver PAWS program, in partnership with the Delta Society, are dedicated to improving quality of life and providing comfort for people on hospice through interaction with trained and registered animals. These animals aren't just dogs and cats: Registered teams (handler and pet) include birds, house rabbits, horses, llamas, and other species. Those assigned to Alzheimer's patients work tirelessly to increase mental awareness through positive animal–human connections. They share love and time with the people who need these the most. The team helps Alzheimer patients change focus, moving it away from themselves and their problems.

The patients often remember pleasant animal experiences from their childhood. Animals create emotional safety and open a channel of nonthreatening communication between patient and team. Animals accept people without qualification or judgment. They don't care how a person looks, what they say, or how they say it. The animals brighten the atmosphere, increasing laughter and play, and decreasing feelings of isolation and fear. When a team is placed with a patient, some people feel spiritual fulfillment or a sense of oneness with life and nature that defies simple explanation.

—MARION NIXON, CREATOR OF PET THERAPY AND VOLUNTEER PROGRAMS

Lucille with Tammy and Gigi – USA
*Tammy and Gigi have brought delight to Alzheimer's patients and hospice residents alike. The most enthusiastic response I saw, however, was from Lucille. As Tammy arrived in her room, she loudly exclaimed "It's a **dog**!" Lucille eagerly awaited their weekly visits until the day she died.*

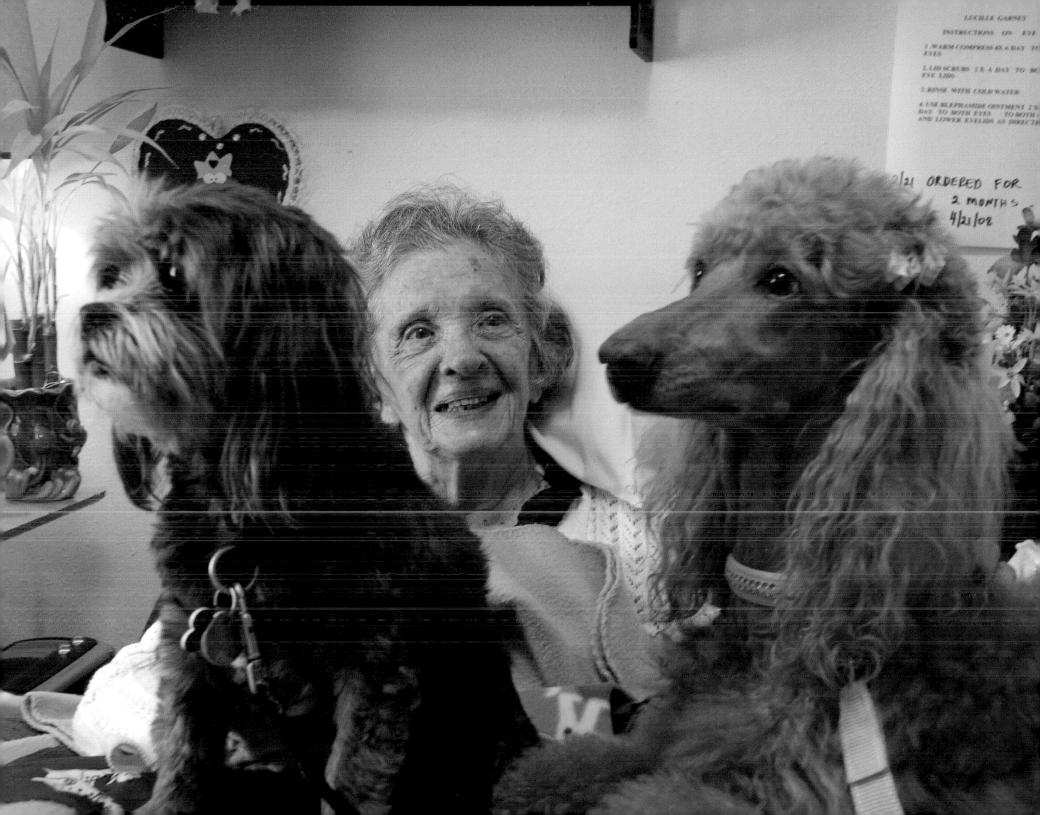

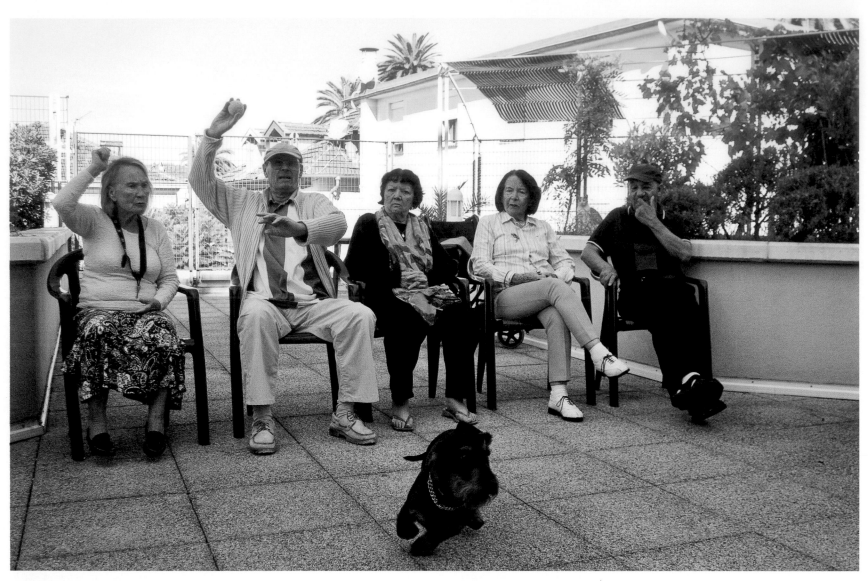

Valerio at the Villa Helios – France

Valerio loves to accompany Elisa when she goes to the Villa Helios, where she is a psychologist and responsible for the day program. Most days he stays quietly in the office, but on Wednesday mornings he helps the residents exercise by chasing balls that they throw for him. He receives treats for his good work, and his presence is a treat for them.

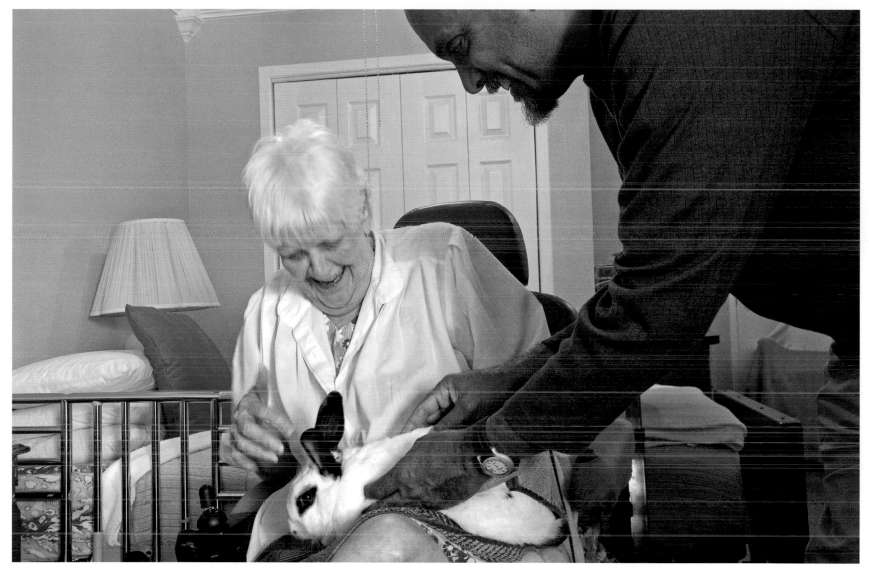

Carmichael presenting Chi to Mavis – USA

When Carmichael learned in a social work class how effective animals could be with ill and dying people, he and Chi, his daughter's rabbit, went for training. This was their first visit to a patient after being certified. Mavis was thrilled with having a soft bunny to caress, and Carmichael was enthusiastic about his new activity. Chi was a success all day and for a long time afterward.

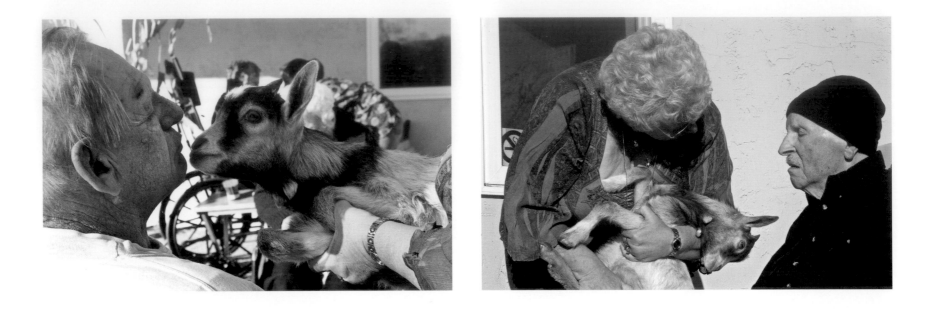

Judy Berry shows off the baby goats at Lakeview Ranch – USA

Most of the residents at Lakeview Ranch were enchanted with the baby goats, while others were not. A disinterested resident one day, however, might be delighted with the animals the next day.

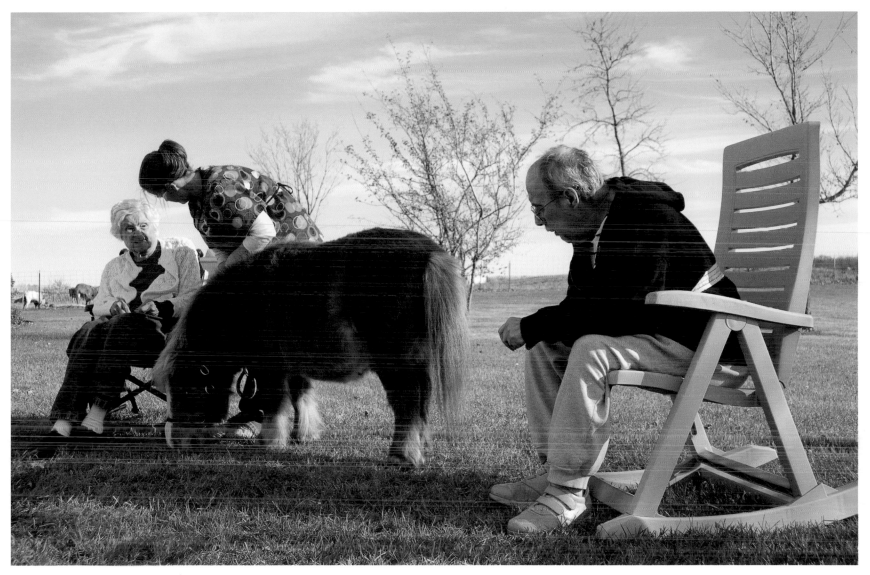

Lakeview Ranch – USA

At Lakeview Ranch in rural Minnesota, several dogs live in two buildings that each house fifteen residents with relatively advanced dementia. More important for many are the farm animals, including a pony, goats, and ducks. Many residents are from farm families.

SIMPLE LESSONS FROM OTHERS' EXPERIENCES

As a student, I worked (mostly by night) in a hospice. There was an old anxious Swiss German lady there, who wandered at night. Once I sat down with her (it must have been around 1:00 AM), took her hands, and prayed with her, though I am an atheist. I can still see her face turning to me and her smile. We remained there a couple of minutes, and she went back with grace to her room.

—ANNE-CLAUDE JUILLERAT, PSYCHOLOGIST

My life with the disease rests on several pillars: The first is maintaining close relationships, for daily connection and basic needs. The second pillar is to seek the help of memory center professionals to assist with comprehension, motivation, and rehabilitation. They can be the most solid allies in preserving a certain degree of autonomy and self-esteem. A professional helped me to relearn how to do simple things that I had forgotten—for example, how to use vending machines, to withdraw money from the ATM, or to organize a diary, all skills taught particularly to meet my needs. I especially found that this training provided me with the support and the motivation necessary to initiate and carry out new projects.

—MARCEL BRASEY, PERSON LIVING WITH THE SYMPTOMS AND DIAGNOSIS OF DEMENTIA, RETIRED BUSINESSMAN

In my long-term-care unit in the university hospital in Nimes, the doors to the nursing station were never closed. Nurses prepared reports and medications while physicians, students, and caregivers met and had informal talks about patients or care. Every day, wandering patients or patients who were feeling lonely enjoyed sitting with us and participating through their presence or with their comments. They could keep talking on their own topics, but most were looking for some interaction, contact, or "a little chat." They were in search of active presence, proximity, and warmth instead of feeling lost in their bedrooms or in the corridors of the unit. This openness to having them with us stopped their incessant wandering for long periods of time, and the encounters always ended in laughter and giggles with the staff.

—FRANÇOISE GUILLO-BEN AROUS, GERIATRICIAN

A few examples of you disabling me—when you honestly believe you are enabling me—are when you pick out "the right clothes" for me, when you speak for me without asking, when you talk about me as if I am not in the room when I am. While I know you intend these to be loving acts, the unintended consequence is to disable me from my own sense of wholeness, my own sense of self-confidence and self-competency. I must always try to deal with the consequences of a failing and faulty set of cognitive skills. You can choose to engage me, to support me, to offer to provide the skills I am missing to complete my task. Or you can do it yourself. It's quicker that way. You can be sure it was done the right way—your way. I need you to honor my way. How do you know what I want to figure out for myself unless you ask me?

—RICHARD TAYLOR, CLINICAL PSYCHOLOGIST;
PERSON LIVING WITH THE SYMPTOMS AND DIAGNOSIS OF DEMENTIA

HELPING CHILDREN UNDERSTAND ALZHEIMER'S DISEASE

When a family member has Alzheimer's disease, it affects everyone in the family, including children and grandchildren. Giving children understandable information about Alzheimer's can help them cope with the disease in their family. The type of relationship the child has with the family member and the child's age are important to help determine:

- what information the child receives
- how the information is presented
- the child's part, if any, in caring for the person with Alzheimer's disease

It is important to answer children's questions simply and honestly. For example, you might tell a young child, "Grandma has an illness that makes it hard for her to remember things."

You can help children know that their feelings of sadness and anger are normal. Comfort them. If children express guilt or feel they may have done something to hurt their grandparent, reassure them that they did not cause the disease.

Do not expect a young child to help care for the person with Alzheimer's disease. Make sure a child of any age has time for her own interests and needs, such as playing with friends, going to school activities, or doing homework. Make sure you spend time with your child, so he does not feel that all your attention is on the person with Alzheimer's.

Help the child understand your own feelings. Be honest about your feelings when you talk with a child, but do not overwhelm her. Many younger children will look to you to see how to act around the person with Alzheimer's. Show children they can still talk with the person, at least in the early stages of the disease. Doing fun things together, with parental supervision depending on the age of the child, can help both the child and the person with Alzheimer's. Here are some things they might do:

- Walk in the neighborhood.
- Do simple arts and crafts.
- Play music, sing.
- Look through photo albums.
- Read stories out loud.

However, in the later stages of disease, the person with Alzheimer's may be completely unresponsive. This may be very hard for a child to understand. Some children might not talk about their negative feelings, but you may see changes in how they act. Problems at school, with friends, or at home can be signs that they are upset. You may want to ask a school counselor or a social worker to help a child understand what is happening and how to cope.

A teenager might find it very hard to accept how the person with Alzheimer's disease has changed. He might find the changes upsetting and not want to be around the older person. It is a good idea to talk with teenagers about their concerns and feelings. Do not force them to spend time with the person who has Alzheimer's. This could make things worse.

If the stress of living with someone who has Alzheimer's disease becomes too great for a child, talk to other family members or friends about helping out. Or find out about, and consider using, respite-care options available in your community. Then both you and your child can get a much-needed break.

—ALZHEIMER'S DISEASE EDUCATION AND REFERRAL CENTER
OF THE NATIONAL INSTITUTE ON AGING

The best way to be a human being is to have a purpose. When you lose your job, when you can't drive, when people begin to stay away from you, even friends and family, when you can't go out by yourself and you find yourself having to adjust your comings and goings to the comings and goings of others—when all this happens almost at once—is it any wonder people with dementia lose their sense of purpose? Everyone, in every shack, hut, home, community, village, city, state, and nation of the world, who is living with dementia is losing or has lost his or her purpose for living. We need your support to redefine our sense of purpose. We need your support to provide opportunities for us to experience what it feels like to be living a purposeful and purpose-filled life every day of our lives.

—RICHARD TAYLOR, CLINICAL PSYCHOLOGIST;

PERSON LIVING WITH THE SYMPTOMS AND DIAGNOSIS OF DEMENTIA

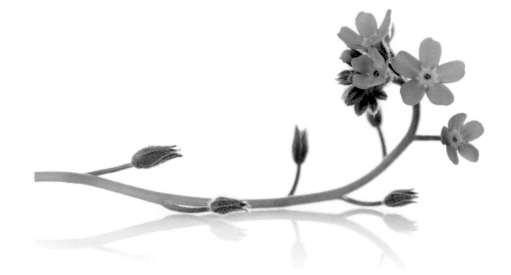

CHAPTER 5

MAINTAINING CAPACITIES

People with dementia are very much living in the present. They have memories of the past, but they may have difficulty accessing them. Some stimuli will help to evoke these, while other memories will remain hidden most of the time. Rather than being "absentminded," they might be thought of as "present-minded, elsewhere" as they get flashes of recall when doing something else. New experiences are often not turned into memories due to brain damage.

Memory clinics, day-care programs, and residential programs encourage reminiscence, which can be triggered by old photographs, familiar objects, and reminders by others of events, people, and accomplishments. People with dementia should not be presented with "Don't you remember . . . ?" or other challenges.

There are many other ways to provide meaningful experiences. The choice begins with knowledge of the individual's past interests and activities. Engaging in familiar activities is important to a sense of well-being and a sense of purpose.

Laura Bramly, an educator, expresses the challenge well:

I firmly believe that one-on-one interaction, or activities that demand interaction from the person with dementia, are what can bring a person with even advanced dementia alive, even temporarily. However, it's ironic that this kind of interaction is lacking in most memory-care facilities. Hence, you end up with lonely seniors lined up in wheelchairs in the hallway or gazing at the T V in the community room.

Generally speaking, life for people with dementia can be so much richer and happier if we stretch our imagination to consider what they are capable of rather than allowing the stigma of dementia to define our perception of their abilities. If we get past the stigma, we realize that it's always possible to build cognitive abilities, and that people have the ability to progress right until the end.

What should we do? Read and cook. Take dictation from a person with dementia and write some postcards to friends and family. Paint, sing songs, play games, recite nursery rhymes, beat a drum, count to a hundred. Find out what the person liked to do! Find a way to help her enjoy the hobbies she used to love. Turn off the @*!# TV, and, for that matter, the radio. Bring some purpose into this person's life. And hug him more and kiss him more, and make sure he has physical contact every day, because this love brings a person with dementia back to the present, or at least makes him present with you in the moment.

People living in the later stages of dementia are living in the present (and by the present, I mean now, this second) because there is nothing else. As a caregiver, you need to step into this reality and realize that all that matters is Right Now, not five minutes ago, and not half an hour from now. If you are able to bring joy into their Right Now, then you have done something wonderful. If, for one second, you were able to make them think, to use their cognitive abilities, to feel curiosity, excitement, wonder, by giving them a gift of any kind, then you have increased the quality of their life for that one second. And because that one second is all that there is, then you have done everything.

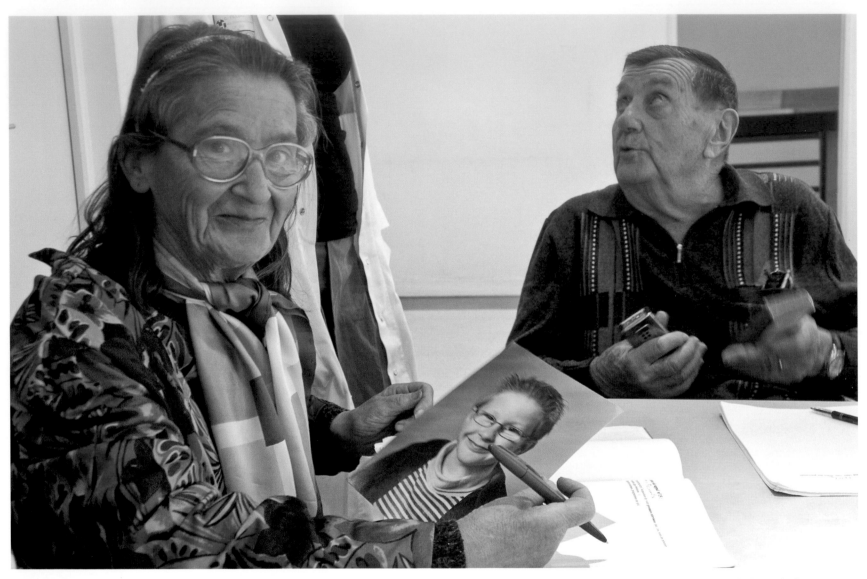

Liliane sharing a photo of her grandson – France

For a reminiscence therapy session at the CMRR memory clinic in Nice, participants were urged to bring in a photo or other item of importance. Many of the photographs were from weddings or trips, but Liliane was delighted to show and discuss the photo of her grandson. Also shown is Jean, a former baker who had played the harmonica all his life, and who entertained the others with some melodies. When he was hit by a car and killed instantly a few weeks after this session, other group members grieved the loss.

A photo may not always be worth a thousand words, but if it stimulates just one great memory it is worth its weight in gold.

—PETER WHITEHOUSE, NEUROLOGIST

Alzheimer's disease is one of the rare illnesses that most touches the identity of the person. With the story of one's life rendered less accessible, projection into the future becomes very difficult. Reminiscence therapy sessions permit the participants to regain the position of a thinking subject. In an environment adapted to their handicap, they can express themselves at the same level as others, an experience that is often no longer the case within the family setting.

—VALERIE LAFONT, SPEECH THERAPIST

People with AD often have lost the key to important parts and episodes of their lives, or they cannot talk about these things. Caregivers and staff members can easily help open the treasure chambers, thus giving comfort and joy. I'll never forget a ninety-five-year-old woman with Alzheimer's whom I often met in the common kitchen of a residential home in Munich, Germany. Most of the time she sat in an old armchair moaning, with a colorful triangular scarf (obviously handmade) on her knees. One day I sat beside her, showing her my knitting work, and at once she stopped moaning and began telling me about her former favorite activity: crocheting. She was beaming as she described how she'd made the scarf years ago. I admired her fine work and she suddenly seemed to straighten her shoulders, being so proud of herself.

—CLAUDIA BAYER-FELDMANN, PSYCHOLOGIST

Major Brami, recipient of five Purple Hearts, in uniform – USA

On November 11, 2007, Veterans Day, a major celebration was held honoring Major Brami for his distinguished twenty-year military career. What was particularly remarkable was that the event was held at the Silverado Senior Living community in Kingwood, Texas, where Major Brami lives. An ROTC group presented the colors, a high school band played, and the major's children and grandchildren were in attendance to hear the Houston mayor's community liaison officer declare the day Major Brami Day. One grandson presented his grandfather with a framed commemorative case he had made that contained all of the major's medals and decorations: five Purple Heart medals, two Bronze Stars, a Bronze Star for valor, three Bronze Stars for combat jumps, Army Commendation Medals, two Combat Infantryman Badges, a Master Parachutist Badge, and numerous others. The Silverado staff always addresses him as "Major Brami," and they take time to listen to him speak about his experiences in World War II and the Korean War. He doesn't usually wear his uniform, but it was normal for him to do so for the visit of a photographer.

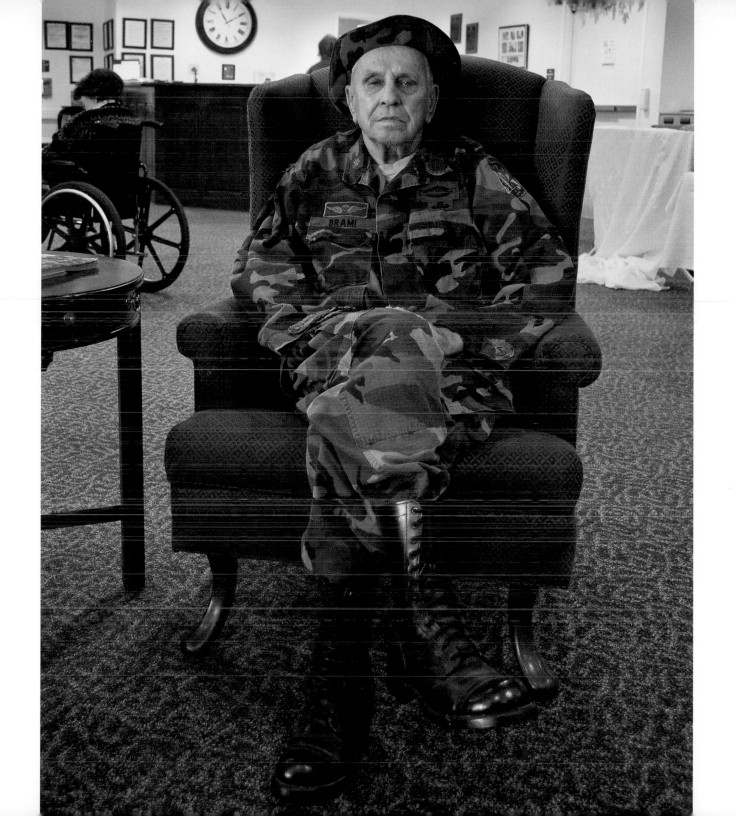

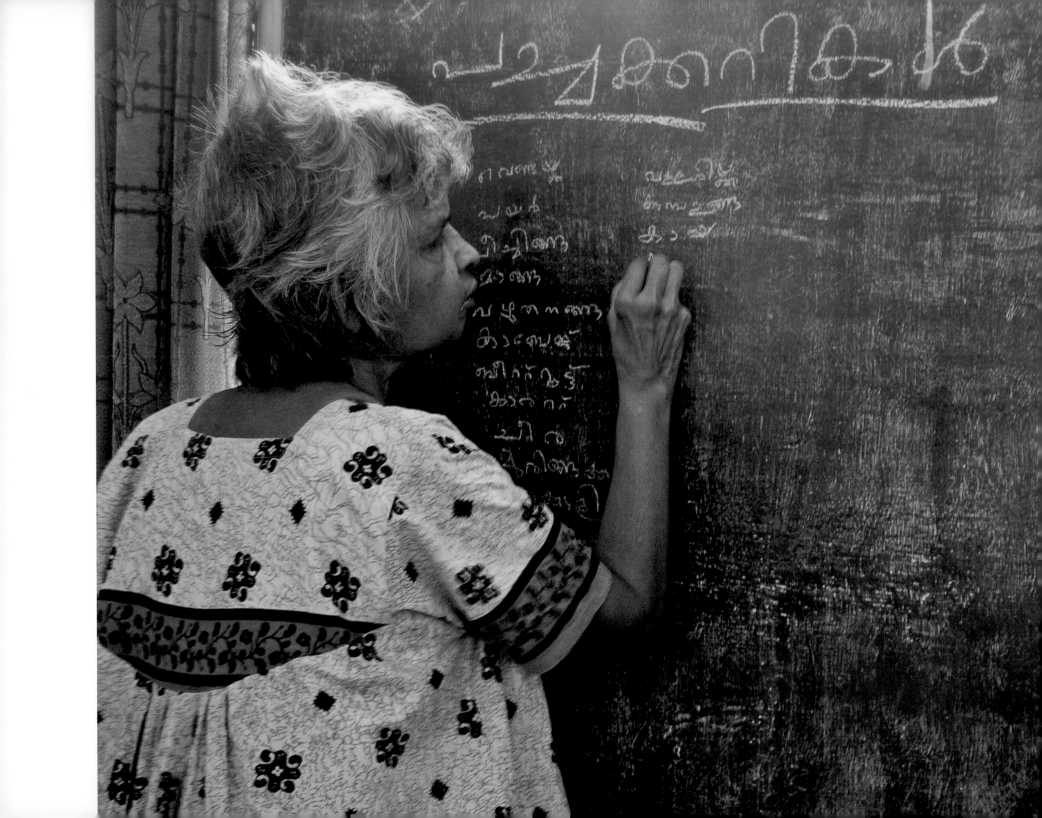

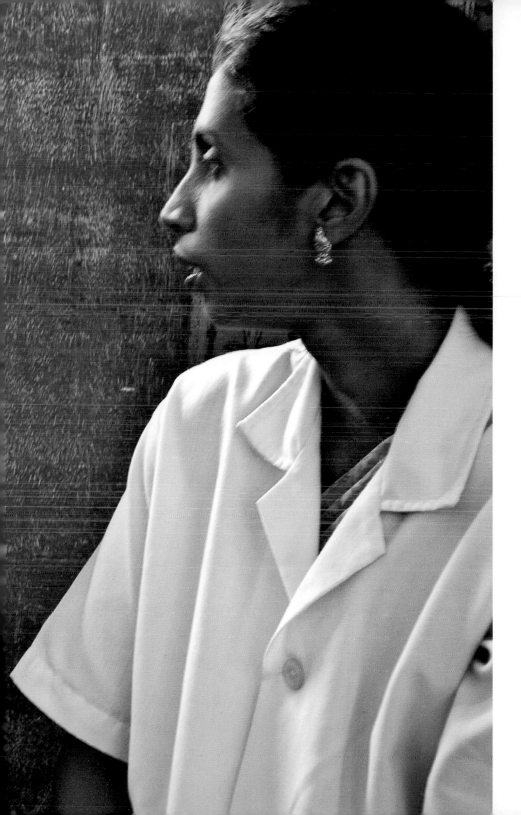

Former math teacher at the blackboard – India

Good care in a group setting involves individualized care. The staff at the day care center in Cochin, India, understands the need to find activities that are meaningful to the participants given both their backgrounds and their present capabilities. This woman, a former mathematics teacher, likes to write numbers on paper or on the blackboard. In such a case, each line is a victory. The center purchased the blackboard to help her feel connected to her past and experience old pleasures. It is a good example of the power of individualized attention in a group setting.

While the subject of this photo is Kay, who is engaged in her book, my clinical eye immediately focused on the woman being fed across the table. When I worked with dementia patients at a nursing facility for veterans, we tried to focus on natural feeding. When a patient began to lose weight and seemed to have what we called poor oral intake—what most would refer to as eating—consideration was always given to the question of whether or not to place a feeding tube. The tube is placed in the stomach to feed a liquid diet, sometimes through the nose and sometimes put through a hole in the stomach through the abdominal wall. It is uncomfortable and can lead to infections or other complications.

As health professionals we often forget that this also deprives people of the simple human act of smelling, tasting, and enjoying food. The problem in most facilities, however, is that to feed a person in the natural way takes time, and staff time is often a valuable and scarce resource. But it can be done. At one facility where I worked, we enlisted volunteers to help feed our residents, and it was wonderful to see them at mealtimes. We had lawyers from downtown in their business suits, older retired veterans who simply wanted to help their fellow vets, young teenagers doing community service through their local high schools. By having them help us feed, we were able to transform a clinical and nutritional need into an opportunity for human interaction. I couldn't have imagined anything that was more important to our residents.

—JUDITH SALERNO, EXECUTIVE OFFICER OF THE U.S. INSTITUTE OF MEDICINE

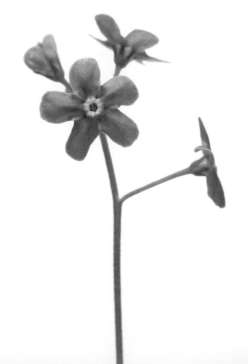

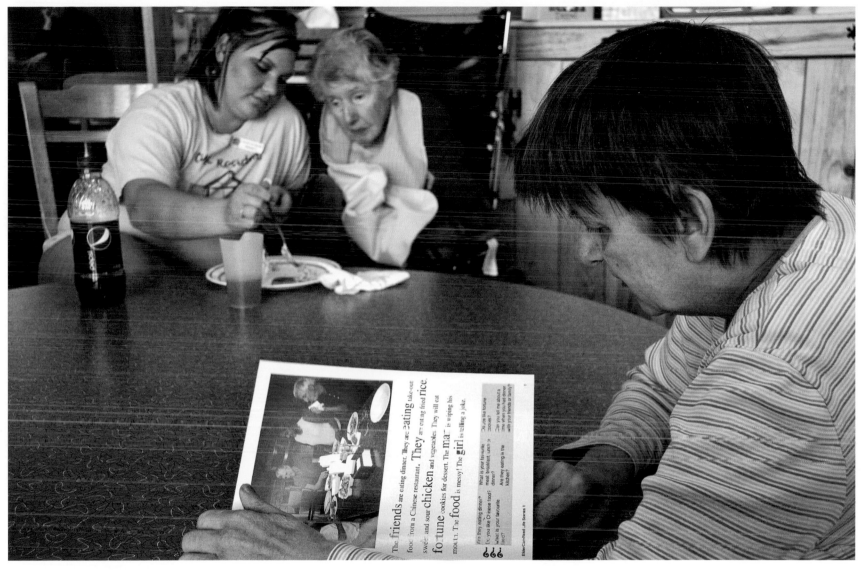

Kay reading the ElderCareRead book – USA

*At Lakeview Ranch in rural Minnesota, one resident, Kay, became intensely interested in Laura Bramly's book, **ElderCareRead: Life Scenes**. Laura had originally created the book for her mother, who at age eighty-five had a stroke that resulted in vascular dementia and significant loss of her memory and cognitive abilities. Laura learned that her mother could still love reading when the material was simplified and the font was larger.*

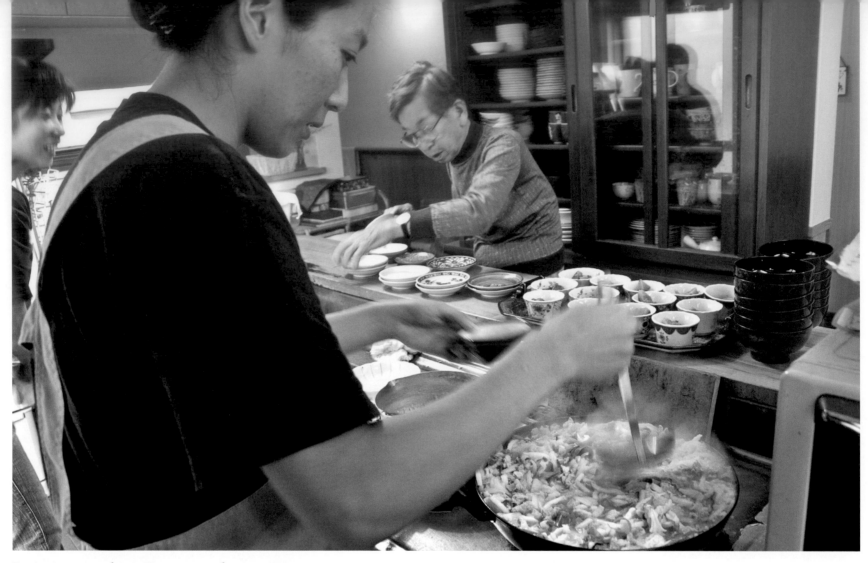

Preparing a meal in a Kyoto group home – Japan

Since there are only nine residents in most Japanese group homes, there is no institutional cooking. Meals are prepared by the staff with assistance from the residents who are able and willing to help. At this group home everyone did something to participate, whether it was laying out the plates and chopsticks or checking on all the dishes to be served, as was the case of the man here, a former chef. Even those with the most limited capacities had a role. Staff and residents then dined together at each meal.

To be of use is to be human. Unfortunately, people with Alzheimer's disease often find themselves in situations that keep them from being useful. Helping them find real ways to be of use is a wonderful contribution. Not only do those with the disease gain a foothold in the real world of social relations, but the people surrounding them feel better, too. Sometimes being of use requires risk—is a cut from using an apple peeler worth the esteem that comes from helping? Each family needs to decide and sometimes needs to sign legal waivers.

—JOAN AMATNIEK, NEUROLOGIST

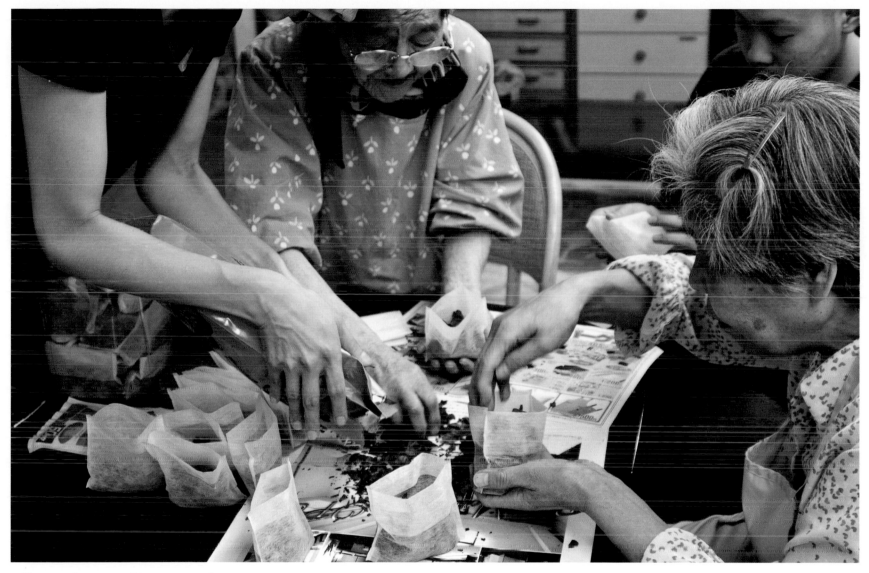

Filling tea bags in a Kyoto group home – Japan
One of the values of activities that are useful and can be done in a group is that by watching others, people can follow the line of action and understand what is needed of them.

Subbamma, eighty-four and diagnosed with Alzheimer's, has been a housewife all her life. She rattles off recipes for the most delectable Indian dishes with the correct ingredients and measures. She helps in sorting out vegetables and performing household chores. Subbamma will make sure that you are well fed and taken care of if you are visiting our center. She is a complete hostess. She had issues with wandering off from her home, but now she has a place to go where she is the hostess—our day center!

—PRIYAMVADA MUDDAPUR, HEALTH-CARE PROFESSIONAL

Subbamma is the prototype of the Alzheimer's patient who has found a meaning within the illness through continuing some of the roles she used to have. She helps in the kitchen, and she makes sure that everybody eats well at the day center she attends, which is what she used to do at home as a housewife while raising her children. She continues her religious practices. When this happens, the symptoms of the illness tend to be more benign and easier to handle.

—DAISY ACOSTA, PSYCHIATRIST

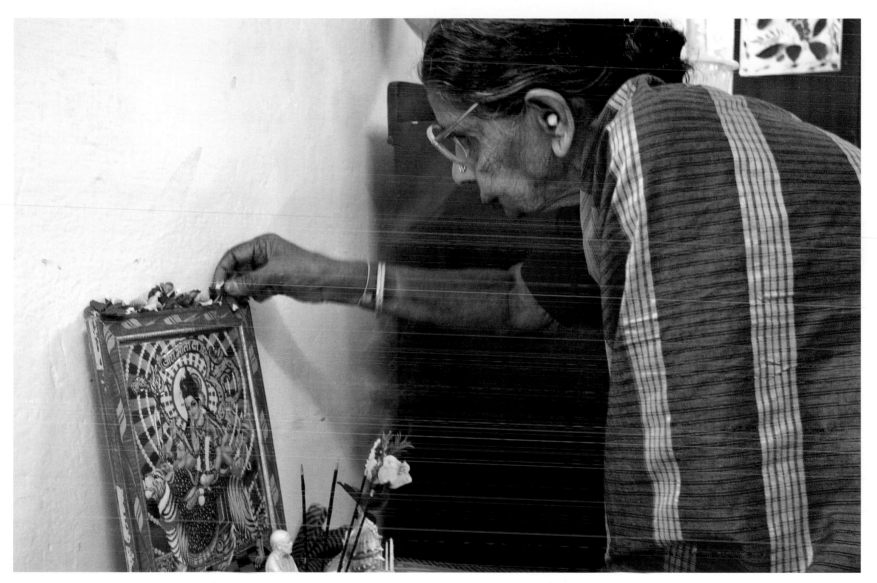

Subbamma's religious ritual – India

Subbamma believes in the power of God and is ready to sing devotional songs any time of the day. She recalls every element of the religious ritual she has been performing for decades, lighting incense and praying to Durga at the day-care center, as well as at home.

Marcel Brasey, a former businessman from Switzerland, describes his self-doubts and the way he has overcome many of them. On his blog and through his public speaking engagements, he has inspired many others.

Am I still competent?

The worst is that I myself used to think that once a person developed Alzheimer's, he was fatally incompetent and hopelessly dependent. Fortunately, in my contacts with other patients at my memory clinic, I could see just the opposite. I now know that we can do a great deal to develop our preserved capacities. If we explore, it's possible to locate these capacities, to bring them into focus, and to separate continued strengths from the forces contributing to our weakness.

The exercise of autonomy is a basic right, especially for a person with memory loss. If it is about the capacity to drive a car, although I cannot do it anymore, my independence wants to say, "I am capable of knowing what is good for me. I can remain like this for a very a long time. Because even if I can hardly explain my reasons, I can still decide! And even if I do not manage to justify my choices, I can still choose!" Here I like to quote Gandhi, who said: "What you do for me, but without me, you do it against me!"

Because the real world passes by too quickly, I rely upon my computer and the Internet. There, I can fully accept myself with the disease. I can read and write at my own speed. The computer allows me the necessary time. It never scolds me, "Hey you've forgotten something!" or "I already told you that!" Even when I make it repeat things ten times, it remains calm and never becomes annoyed. It accepts me as I am. It's like a friend—almost human—and at any rate it has become indispensable in helping me to live with the disease.

I face a demanding task. The forced abandonment of my profession came as an enormous shock. How can anyone fill this void? The English website http://dasninternational.org is a place where young patients in early stages can talk about the challenges of living with dementia. The site encouraged me to create my own French version—http://survivre-alzheimer.com. There I write about various aspects of my situation, which I then share with others in the same situation. This space enables me to feel useful and to emphasize the capacities that remain within me. I also use my site to remain connected with my family and friends. It has become another way of helping them understand and appreciate my handicaps and hopes.

—MARCEL BRASEY, LIVING WITH THE DIAGNOSIS AND SYMPTOMS OF DEMENTIA,
RETIRED BUSINESSMAN

MONTESSORI METHODS FOR PEOPLE WITH DEMENTIA

Some of the most interesting work I know concerning the maintenance of capacities has been done by Cameron Camp and others who have been inspired by his writings and talks.

Maria Montessori was an advocate of human rights. Every Montessori educator and trainer I've met agrees: "Providing respect and dignity to the individual is the most important thing." Her educational program for children was based on clinical observation and the application of rehabilitation techniques to the process of learning, but its creation was driven by a passion to give all children a chance to have a valued role in society.

In this way she provided technologies and a moral imperative that have immediate relevance for the way we think about and deal with dementia. For example, one of her key lessons for Montessori teachers was "Never speak ill about a child in front of the child—nor when the child is absent." That lesson translates most poignantly into how we treat those with dementia.

We have used the Montessori Method as the inspiration for creating meaningful activities and social roles for people with dementia. One example is intergenerational programming, where older adults with dementia serve as teachers or mentors to preschool children in one-on-one interactions. They can teach children how to fold or hang up clothes, use tools, count, or set a table.

The key is to first make sure that the people with dementia can perform the teaching activity, then provide them with practice, and then let them work with children. Our training seminars show that people with dementia can learn new procedures and get better at them over time. If we look at their strengths rather than their deficits and provide appropriate support and opportunities for new learning, we begin to view these men and women in a new light.

Another example is when we have trained people with dementia to become group activity leaders for others similarly diagnosed. This is directly translated from Montessori classrooms, where older children present lessons to younger children. In our case, we have trained men and women with dementia to lead reading and discussion groups composed entirely of their peers.

Other examples of basic Montessori principles in action include:

- *using templates (for instance, using an outline of a table setting as a guide to placing items)*
- *using large, thick print with high contrast to its background*
- *matching your own speed of movement to the person with dementia's*
- *demonstrating clearly what the person with dementia should do before assigning a task*
- *giving choices ("this or that" choices, not "what would you like" options, are usually best)*
- *asking the opinion of those with dementia*
- *providing an environment that demands acknowledging everyone involved as a human being*

—CAMERON CAMP, PSYCHOLOGIST

If you are caring for someone with Alzheimer's, you will need to go into their world—the Alzheimer's World—in order to maintain your own sanity and well-being.

In the Alzheimer's World, communication is very different than in the real world. For me, there is only one other person in the Alzheimer's World most of the time—my mother. One thing that makes my mother different from the rest of us is that her short-term memory is gone. It would be foolish of me to expect her to remember what I said a little while ago. She can't.

As Alzheimer's progresses, short-term memory disappears. It no longer exists. Once you accept and understand that short-term memory is gone, you should not be surprised if those with Alzheimer's ask the same questions repeatedly. They can't remember if they asked you a question—once or ten times. You can remember because you are still in the real world. Your short-term memory is still working.

As I thought about this, I came to a simple conclusion. Instead of trying to change the Alzheimer's World, instead of trying to fight it, not only would I accept it as a reality, I would go into it and learn how to communicate effectively.

If you try this, you will start feeling good about yourself, and soon the person who has Alzheimer's will start feeling pretty good also. Instead of sending a nasty vibe, you will be sending a very different signal—I care. You will be doing something that is important: creating an environment that is safe and secure. Once Alzheimer's patients start feeling safe and secure, they become kinder and more gentle.

—BOB DEMARCO, FOUNDER/EDITOR, THE ALZHEIMER'S READING ROOM

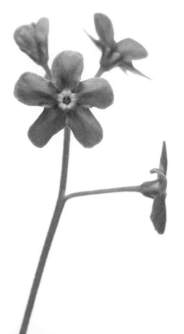

CHAPTER 6

IMPROVING COMMUNICATION

As Alzheimer's disease progresses, expressing oneself verbally often becomes harder. The right words may not come easily to patients with cognitive challenges. The difficulty of making a clear statement is frustrating for them. Caregivers often become frustrated as well, and their impatience compounds the issues. Even when the words themselves are clear, the thoughts behind them may be confused or unrelated to the present situation. The temptation to try to drag the person into "our reality" is great, but challenging them worsens the problem. People who have spoken a second language for many years may forget it in the late stages of their illness, reverting to their native language, which others in their social circle may not know.

The good news is that there are more effective communication approaches that all of us can learn. These also help reduce incidents of aggressive behavior. Judy Berry, founder and director of an Alzheimer's care facility, provides this sound advice:

For me, it is instructive to reverse the conventional communication paradigm and to look out through the eyes of the patient. If I were the patient, how would I want to be treated? In order to communicate effectively, you need to not only listen, but also take cues from nonverbal behavior, to learn by trial and error what words and actions work. Try. Keep trying. It takes a serious effort all the time, every day. If you accomplish this mission, you will improve the quality of life of the person suffering from dementia and your own quality of life. Instead of feeling that you are surrounded by four very high walls, you might finally see that there is a door in the room. Why not walk through the door?

SOUND ADVICE AND TIPS FROM INDIVIDUALS WITH EARLY MEMORY LOSS

- *Speak with a smile, so I know that you care. If you are tense, remember that I feel your tension, too. A smile takes away tension and helps put me at ease.*
- *Use language I understand and keep it simple, without jargon or slang. Rephrase information if I'm having trouble understanding.*
- *Slow down your speech. Keep it short and to the point, one idea at a time. Be clear and concise.*
- *Let me take the time to think through what you've said to me. It takes me extra time to think through the meaning of words.*
- *Let me set the pace of the conversation. Let me take charge and be the leader.*
- *Make sure you have my attention.*
- *Pause once you say your thoughts. Give me time to find the words and to say my thoughts.*
- *Ask me questions to help me find the words. Please repeat information if I ask.*
- *Make sure I hear you. Ask if I understand what you have said. Adjust the tone of your voice and remember, louder is not always better.*
- *Face me when you talk; eye contact helps to get my complete attention.*
- *Please be patient! Don't give up on me! I really do want to be a part of the conversation.*

The biggest obstacle in connecting with people with dementia is our own ego. So much of our habitual way of communicating with others is based on this simple, unspoken agreement: "I'll reflect you back to you, if you'll reflect me back to me." It takes a lot of cognitive finesse to keep this game going, and people with irreversible dementia are eventually unable to play it with us. When this happens, when they cease to reflect our ego-images back to us in our interactions with them, we say they are "gone."

One way to make the "gone" reappear is for scientists to find a cure for their disappearance. Another way for the "gone" to reappear is for our egos to disappear when we communicate with people with dementia.

Here is a simple way we can do this—intellectually simple but emotionally very difficult. The next time you communicate with someone who is not at his or her cognitive best, remind yourself of this: "This interaction is not about me. This interaction is about someone who is seeking connections on terms that may not advance the interests or needs of my ego. I am going to go where your needs are taking you. I am going to be with you in that place, wherever and however it is. I am going to let my ego disappear now. I am going to love you in your image instead of trying to re-create you in mine."

That is the cure to Alzheimer's disease in the present; that is the great medicine that will make the "gone" reappear. The world is face-to-face with a reality to which only our own spiritual maturity can meaningfully respond. Either we learn how to love each other, or we keep disappearing to each other.

—MICHAEL VERDE, PRESIDENT, MEMORY BRIDGE, CHICAGO, ILLINOIS, USA

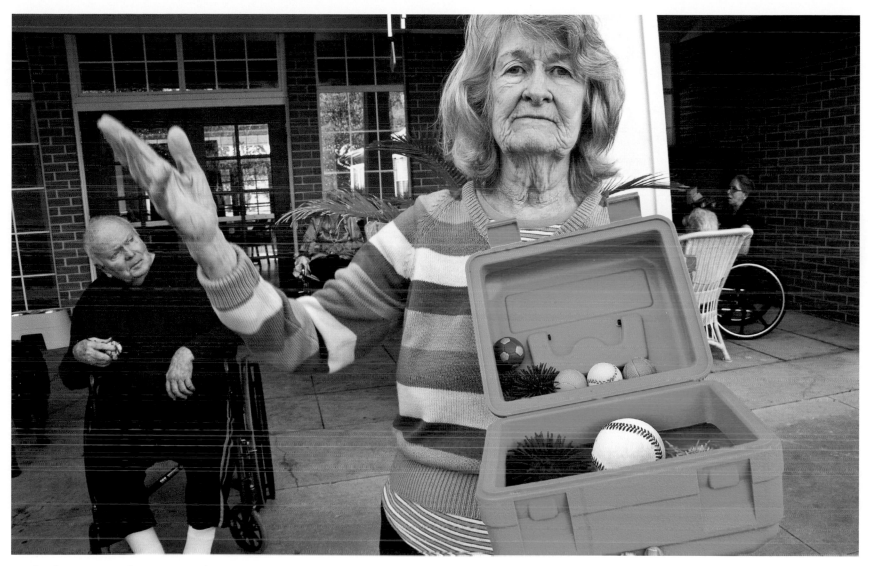

Rachael presenting her treasure box – USA

Rachael remained very spirited despite her growing cognitive difficulties. When she saw I was willing to listen and ask questions, she spent fifteen minutes telling me the name and story of each of the "occupants" of her treasure box. At the end, when she exclaimed, "God bless America!" I took this photo.

I had a good time with her. I could not have done this a few years ago, before I was taught by many wonderful caregivers how to let go of my reality and go into another's. I wish I had known how to do this when my maternal grandparents lived with Alzheimer's and I too often fell silent in their company.

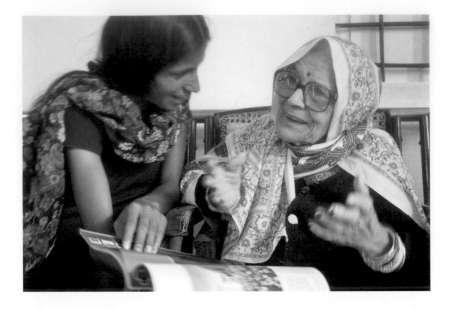
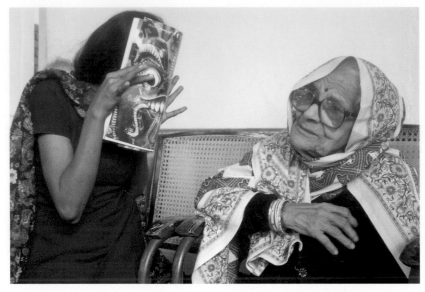

Indian philosophy has always spoken of impermanence, of the here and now, of living in the present or in the moment, and of being thankful for whatever you have. One disease that makes a person experience all of the above is dementia. When I first started as a care manager, I realized that we take a lot of things for granted, not thinking about them, just as we chew our food the moment it is put into our mouths. When I saw that I had to prompt my patients every time a morsel was placed in their mouths, I started appreciating every little bit of life. Being able to see, communicate, eat, sleep, relate to other human beings—these became my reasons to be thankful. Anyone who knows this disease or who has experienced caregiving probably has developed an attitude of gratitude.

With dementia, you lose parts of the person's capacities bit by bit. But there is so much life left and it is up to us to cash it in. I see some of my clients—men and women who led successful lives—now throwing tantrums when eating or insisting on doing an activity over and over again, asking questions repeatedly. But I also find that they are often nonjudgmental, loving, caring, and as pure as snow. They reciprocate love. They are perfect sounding boards. They give back what you offer to them. No guru has taught me so much as they have taught me and I bless them. Being with them, I am reminded of the impermanence of life. I express my love to them every single day.

—PRIYAMVADA MUDDAPUR, HEALTH-CARE PROFESSIONAL

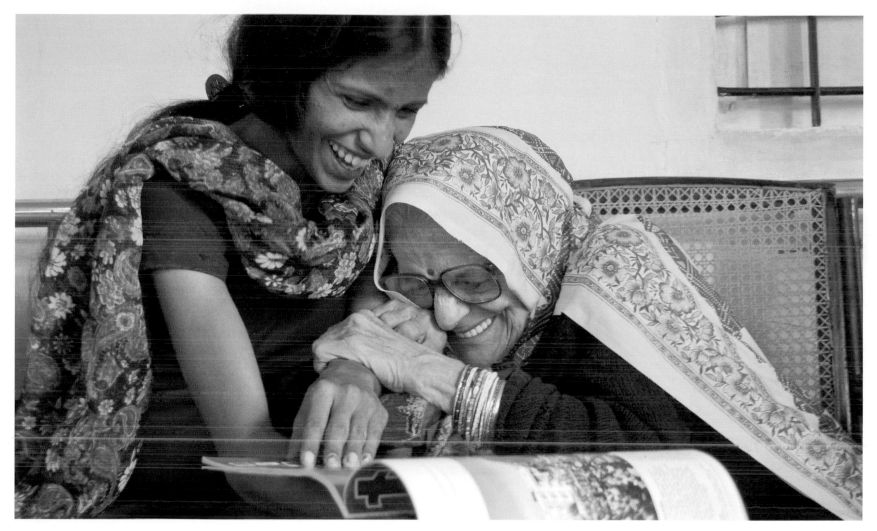

Reading with a caregiver can alleviate the boredom of memory loss. Even when words lack meaning, the act engages and can provoke conversation. An astute caregiver flexibly transitions to other activities, in this case peek-a-boo, a game played across all cultures from early infancy.

—JOAN AMATNIEK, NEUROLOGIST

Ashwani and Didi – India

When Didi came to the Bangalore Nightingales day care center, she was extremely depressed, lonely, wheelchair-bound, and on a catheter. Now she is free of the catheter, walks with minimal assistance, and is one of the most cheerful and sociable participants, appreciative for the loving attention of Ashwani, Dr. Priyamvada, and other staff.

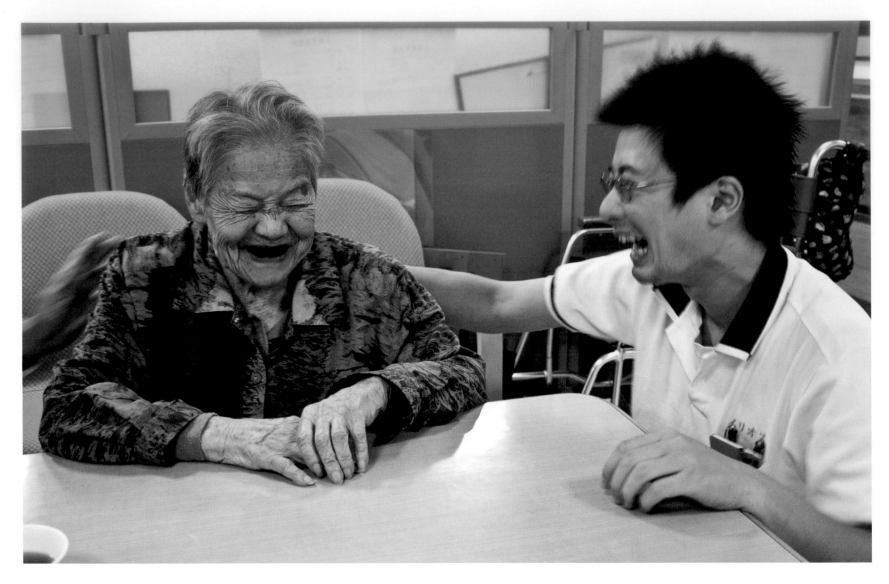

Laughter from the heart – Japan

This aide in an Alzheimer's unit in Kyoto knew how to bring good humor, laughter, and an elevation of mood to the people he worked with. Looking at the photo, Françoise Guillo-Ben Arous commented, "Who is the happiest? Laughing erases everything. Patients connect more easily, and laughter keeps illness away for both caregivers and patients."

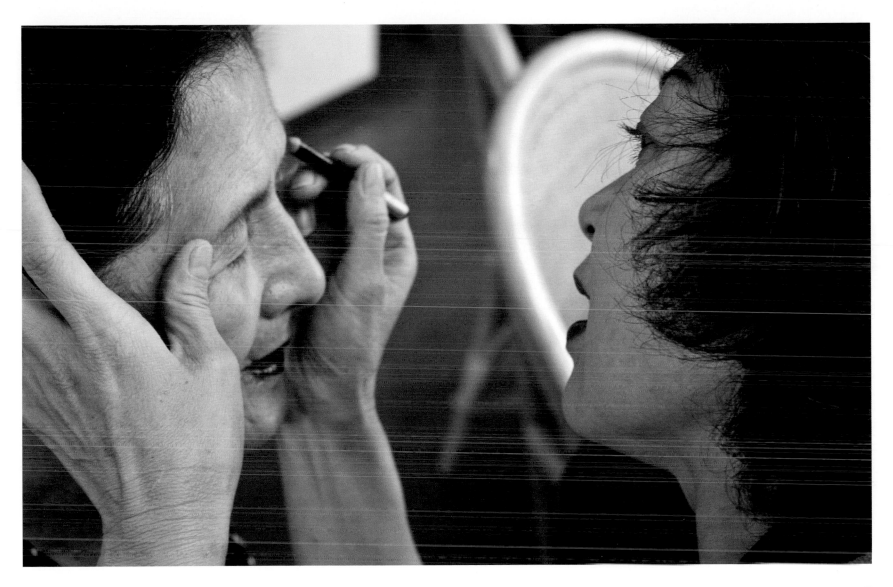

Makeup session before an excursion – Japan

When the director of this Kyoto group home announced to the nine residents that they were going on an excursion to a local temple, she added, "So you all have to look your best." She then brought out a small box of makeup and for the next hour put eyeliner, lipstick, and rouge on each of the seven women who would be going out. They were all delighted to have this attention and to see the results of her efforts in the mirror. The director joked that it was "Makeup Therapy."

How can I tell him?
Occasionally he comes
and sits by me, holds my hand,
speaks in tones I can trust.
Sometimes he sings to me.
and the strangest thing
he does is to get up close
and match his breaths to mine.

I need him here always
but he comes and goes.

I ought to make the most
Of the little he gives me,
But I don't know how.
I try to blink, smile,
Move my limbs, but I can't
Be sure he sees or understands.
Maybe he'll not come back.
How can I tell him?

—John Killick, excerpt from
"Getting Through (1)," Dementia Diary: Poems and Prose

Livia in the beauty salon – USA

At the time of this photo, Livia had advanced Alzheimer's disease and was placed on hospice at the Heather Hill Hospital Alzheimer's unit. Livia no longer recalled English, though she had spoken it for the half century since she'd become a US resident. Her husband, her children, and the staff did not speak Latvian, the language of her childhood, and they didn't understand her when she spoke it. Livia received a great deal of nonverbal communication, however, in the form of hugs and a daily beauty salon visit to assure her that she was still valued. She died a short time later.

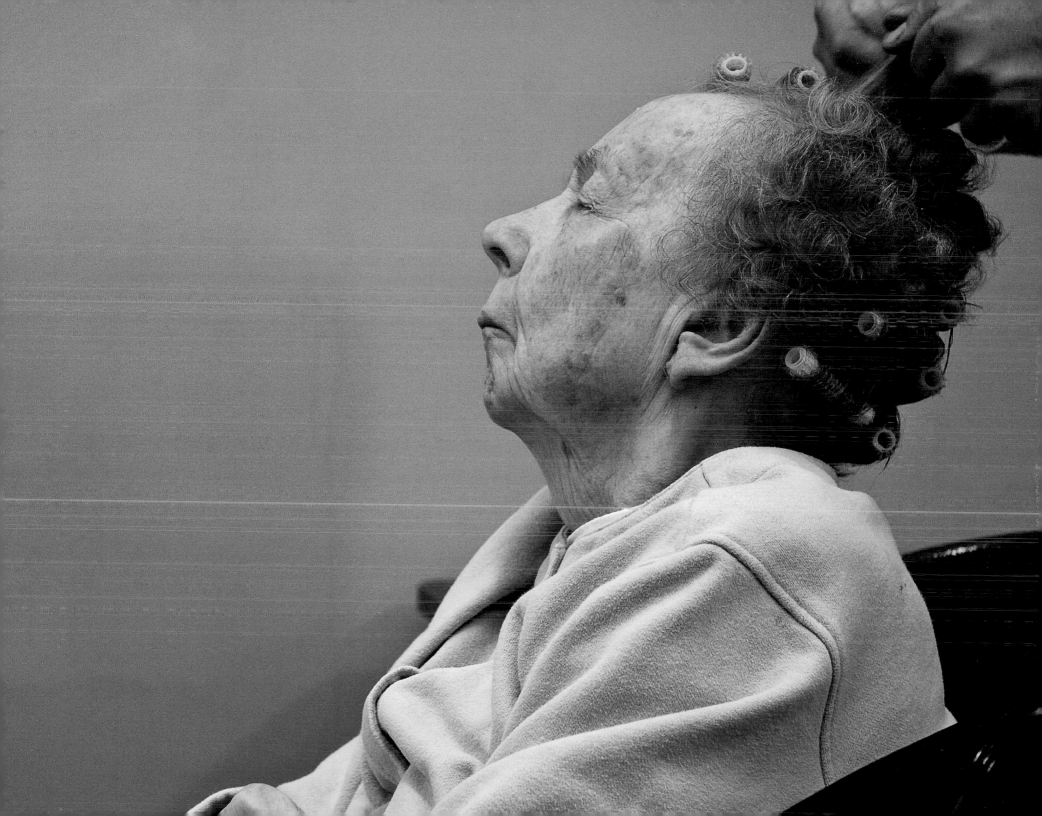

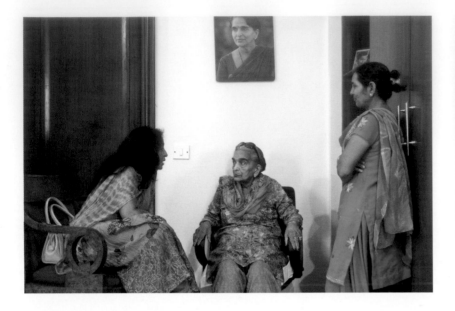 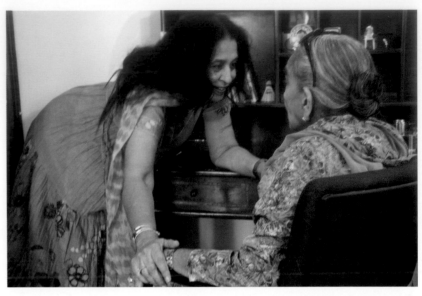

Renu and Mrs. Kumar – India

*Renu works as a volunteer with the Delhi chapter of the Alzheimer's and Related Disorders Society of India (ARDSI). She explained that her ARDSI training has helped her to reach out to and connect with her first cousin, fifteen years her senior. Although Mrs. Kumar seems not to recognize her son or other family members, Renu comes very close, touches her cousin's hand or arm, maintains strong eye contact, and smiles while speaking about things she remembers. "Usually after about fifteen minutes, something I say triggers her recognition of who I am, and with that recognition comes a strong emotional reaction. Then she speaks with me in an animated fashion for a few minutes, before slipping away, back into her isolation." This is **exactly** what happened when I accompanied her the next day to photograph.*

Other people who work with Naomi Feil's Validation Therapy techniques have had dramatic breakthroughs using compassionate touch, behavioral mirroring, and a deep connection between the patient and the practitioner.

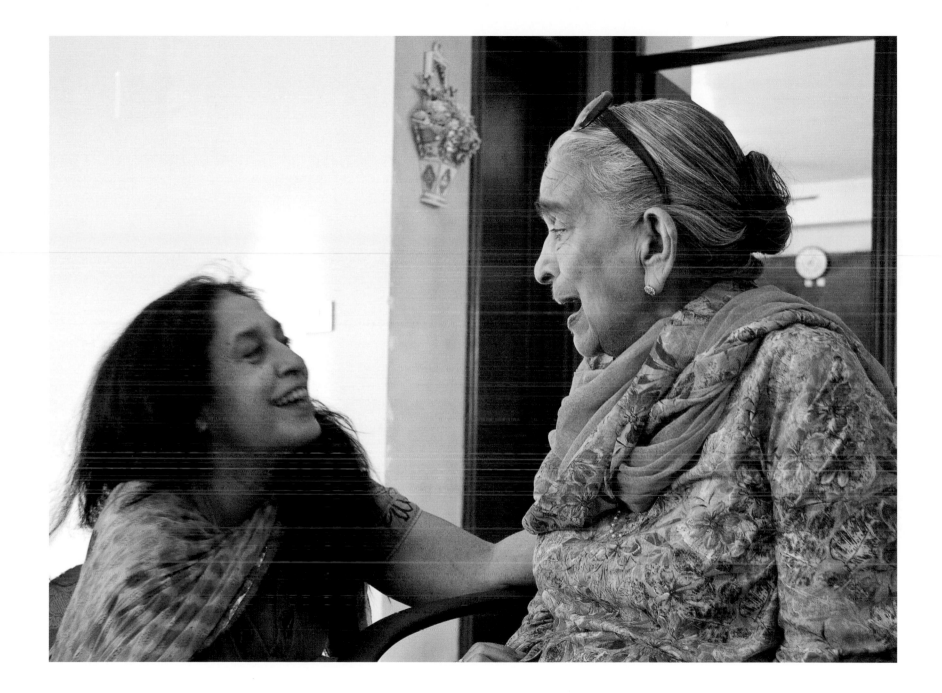

Everyone around us lovingly wants us to be who we were. They understood us then. They knew us then. They could connect with us then. But what about today? Who enables me to stay in today? This day, my day, your day, is all the day we have to live in together right now.

Living in today is easier for you. It comes naturally. Living in today is difficult for me. I do not always understand what is going on around me, or in me. I forget and get confused about parts of today, even before the sun goes down. Today is always a partial mystery to me. Is it any wonder I pull into myself, withdraw, and become paranoid and defensive?

Help me understand today, every day, maybe even twice a day, or thirty times a day. Always introduce yourself. Ask me if I know, or want to know, why you are here, what you are going to do, where I am being taken, why I am going there, how long I'll be, what happens after that. Tell me the day, the date, the season, something about the weather. Engage me. When you assume I do not need to know, when you act as if my knowing is not your most important priority, when you act this way it sends an unintended disabling message to me. It tells me my needs come second to yours.

—RICHARD TAYLOR, CLINICAL PSYCHOLOGIST;
PERSON LIVING WITH THE SYMPTOMS AND DIAGNOSIS OF DEMENTIA

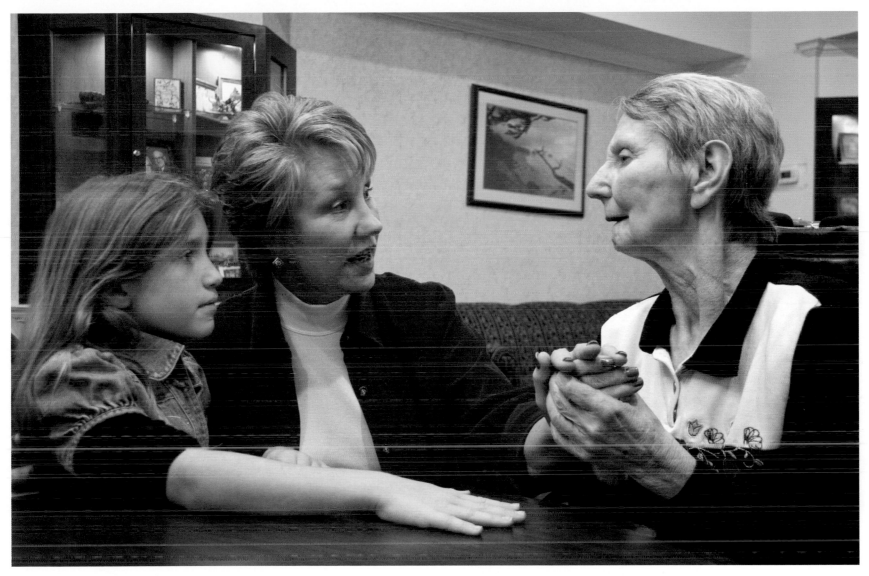

Daphne and Margie, helped to connect by Lara – USA

Daphne and her grandmother Lara visited Lara's mother, Margie, for the Thanksgiving celebration at the Silverado Senior Living Alzheimer's community in Cypresswood, Texas. Daphne was saddened by her great-grandmother's loss of verbal communication skills, but responded to Lara's questions about the piano recital she would give the next day. After Daphne finished speaking, Margie signaled with some noises that she had heard her great-granddaughter's story.

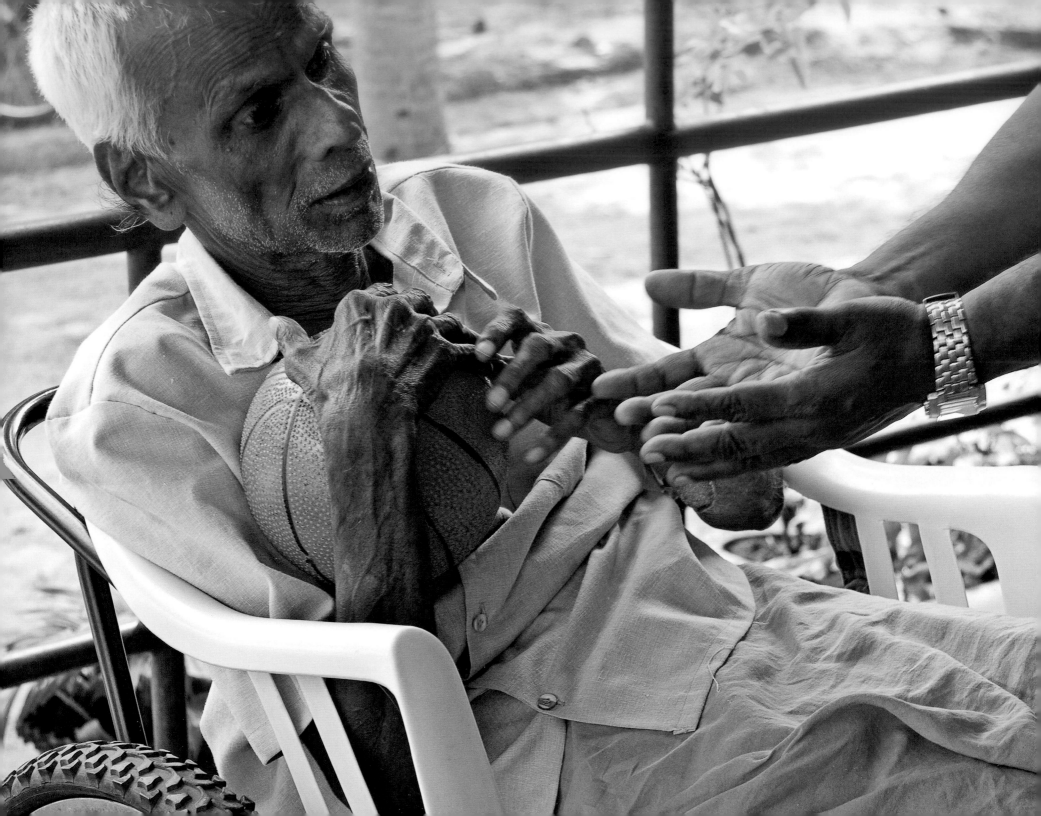

When people with Alzheimer's or related disorders keep a firm hold on things or other people—especially in the later stages of the disease—we should bear in mind that they have experienced many losses so far. They've lost abilities, they've lost friends, and they've lost a great deal of their self-esteem. So let them hold on to balls, dolls, stuffed animals, blankets, our warm hands, or whatever they need.

—CLAUDIA BAYER-FELDMANN, PSYCHOLOGIST

"May we have your ball, please?" – India
This man's guarding of the ball during an exercise period brought kind requests to return it to the group, not chastisement.

"WANDERING"? NO, SEARCHING

Wandering is one of the strangest behavioral disturbances in AD. The biological origin of the symptom remains unclear, but between 15 and 50 percent of patients at an advanced stage of the disease will experience incessant walking during the day or night. This symptom often occurs in association with agitation, disorientation, and anxiety. The patients may fall, or be hurt. They often try to escape from nursing care facilities or from their homes, either alone or by following visitors as they depart. They can look restless and anxious. Patients can walk for hours inside a home or a nursing care facility and stop only when exhausted.

They seem to be looking for something or somebody. In a symbolic way, this incessant marching can be perceived as a quest. We are tempted to find a reason, and sometimes there is one for this apparently aimless wandering. I have seen patients trying to return to their former residence, or to any place to which they have a strong affective link. Others show a different pattern of wandering: Some insist on standing up and starting to explore exits many times in a day, or only during the night.

This is always very stressful for the family and caregivers, who feel that their loved one will be endangered or lost. So what can we do? The priority is to make everything safe for the people and allow them the freedom to move and walk as far as possible in an adapted and secure environment. The space should include architectural constraints. We should also try to provide pleasant physical activities and the presence of others. Accompany them for a walk if possible at dedicated moments in the day. Be aware of the high risk of fall, and adapt the diet to account for increased activity.

—FRANÇOISE GUILLO-BEN AROUS, GERIATRICIAN

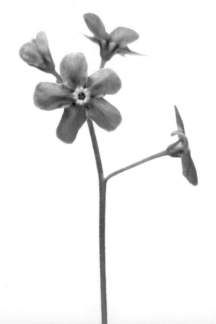

CHALLENGING BEHAVIORS

Aggressive behavior by Alzheimer's patients can cause enormous stress for everyone concerned. The fact that I saw almost none of it in any of my visits has a simple explanation: Knowledgeable caregivers understand that the way to manage challenging behavior is to prevent it in the first place, and they know how to do so. Steve Winner offers insights into the problem and the solution at the Silverado residential communities. The chart on the next two pages is a translation of a flyer prepared by Philippe Robert, Valerie Lafont, and Julie Piano at the Center for Memory Resources and Research of Nice, which also offers sound advice.

Since we founded Silverado Senior Living in 1996, we have sought to serve the most vulnerable persons with dementia—those who exhibit dangerous or destructive behaviors. Assisting someone with memory deficiencies is very difficult as they move through increasing stages of debilitation. Add significant behavior challenges, and care support can become totally overwhelming.

Persons with behavior issues in addition to dementia are often more isolated, restricted, and restrained. They are frequently overmedicated with multiple drugs that have been added upon one another over time. At some point no one can be sure if the medications are helping or indeed causing the behavior.

Many environments and programs that serve people with dementia are inappropriate for the task, with staff members who are not sufficiently trained to prevent aggressive behavior. At these places, when a behavior problem is generated, the resident is often asked to leave.

Finding a new home can be difficult and traumatic. Too often, people with behavioral issues are moved to a place that restrains them physically, often by using larger doses of behavior-controlling medications. Many continue to believe this is all that can be done.

Silverado provides environments designed to assist our residents in having more freedom by reducing fear, confusion, and frustration. Residents are assessed by our RN directors of health services, with input from physician medical directors, to ensure that medications are reviewed and possibly reduced. Potential pain or depression symptoms are diagnosed and treated, generally reducing or eliminating behavior issues. Our associates receive extensive training in behavior management and prevention. Treating residents with dignity and respect, giving them time to understand and perform tasks, using validating communication, and offering many opportunities for choice, recognition, and self-expression all help allay resident fear and reduce frustration. The result is far fewer behavior issues.

Once medical problems are managed and residents receive appropriate support and communication, we deal with the last significant creator of inappropriate behavior: boredom. People with dementia are no different from the rest of us. When we have too much time on our hands, we tend to get into trouble. Silverado provides environments full of life, with pets, children, and age-appropriate engagement activities throughout the day and evening. Our right living environments, expert medical support, trained and experienced associates, along with person-centered programs and support, have allowed us to radically reduce negative behaviors. The result is a notably enhanced quality of life for our residents and their families.

—STEPHEN WINNER, HEALTH-CARE PROFESSIONAL

CHALLENGING BEHAVIORS
Things to do and not to do in various situations

Opposition: Refusal of Care	Aberrant Motor Behavior	Agitation
To Do: 1. Be kind and adapt your behavior 2. Try to put the caregiving aside for as long as possible 3. Listen carefully and take the time to know the reason for the refusal 4. Ask for help from the patient, privileging his/her autonomy 5. Ask another staff member to take over the caregiving 6. Negotiate in order to assure the priority care tasks	**To Do:** 1. Verify whether s/he is wearing appropriate walking shoes 2. Facilitate the resident's strolling while watching out to assure the general security and well-being of other residents 3. Assure that there is a regular presence of someone with the resident 4. Walk with the resident and accompany him to his room or to the living room	**To Do:** 1. Be kind 2. Use contact, touch, hugs, sing a song 3. Be reassuring, offer security 4. Try to discuss and re-orient the resident toward another idea 5. Make a diversion 6. Propose an activity or a walk 7. Establish daily routines 8. Find a way around moments of fatigue or nervousness 9. Limit the number or length of visits 10. Assure a permanent presence after sunset 11. Isolate the patient
Not to Do: 1. Infantilize 2. Moralize to the patient 3. Speak in an authoritarian manner 4. Reprimand 5. Force the resident 6. Use contentious means	**Not to Do:** 1. Put a barrier in the route, stop him from advancing 2. Require him to sit, even during meals 3. Leave obstacles in the pathway (damp floor, etc.) 4. Leave doors to technical spaces open 5. Leave the doors permitting access to outside open	**Not to Do:** 1. Have brutal reactions, or return the aggression (you need to keep your cool) 2. Generate an anxiety-inducing ambience (noise, light, etc.) 3. Appeal in an incessant manner 4. Use contentious means

In Every Case: Verify at the outset that the appearance of behavioral problems is not the result of a somatic problem or of an environmental cause. Change the circumstances that lead to the appearance of a behavioral problem. Know the usual personality of the resident as well as his or her history. **Agitation/Aggression is an urgent situation where every other activity must stop.**

Aggression	Delirium, Hallucinations	Screaming
To Do: 1. Be kind. 2. Use contact, touch, hugs, sing a song. 3. Be reassuring, offer security. 4. Try to discuss and reorient the resident toward another idea. 5. Create a diversion. 6. Propose an activity or walk. 7. Propose a snack or a light drink. 8. Remove dangerous objects. 9. Ensure a secure perimeter. 10. Ask for help if needed. 11. Isolate the patient. 12. Call the doctor.	To Do: 1. Indicate to the resident that we don't hear/see what she hears/sees, but that we believe her 2. Use reassuring words and phrases 3. Try to change the conversation, to orient the resident to another idea 4. If the problem triggers fear, intervene to assure the protection of the resident and those around her 5. Assure a regular presence 6. Call the doctor	To Do: 1. Speak 2. Gain eye contact 3. Hold his hand 4. Create a soothing, relaxed ambience 5. Propose a snack or a light drink
Not to Do: 1. Have brutal reactions, or return the aggression (keep your cool). 2. Generate an anxiety-inducing ambience (noise, light, etc.). 3. Feel hurt by what the patient says. 4. Increase his fear. 5. Infantilize the patient. 6. Adapt a superior or authoritarian tone. 7. Try to reason with the patient. 8. Make humiliating remarks, humiliate. 9. Punish. 10. Use contentious means.	Not to Do: 1. Panic 2. Try to reason with the resident 3. Infantilize or ridicule 4. Deny the delirium 5. Hold a conversation about the delirium 6. Create complex and ambiguous situations 7. Use contentious means	Not to Do: 1. Cry louder than the resident (don't try to cover the voice of the resident) 2. Generate an anxiety-inducing ambience (light, noise . . .) 3. Minimize the pain 4. Use contentious means

—*Philippe Robert, Valerie Lafont, and Julie Piano, from an EHPAD pamphlet, translated from French*

This letter came to me from someone who was moved by a photograph that appeared in my earlier book, *Alive with Alzheimer's*. I treasure the letter. I hope you will be inspired by the images in this chapter to sing, hum, play CDs, bring your instrument on a visit, prepare and gift a personalized playlist on an iPod—whatever works for you and your loved one.

Dear Cathy,

My mother died in March, and I was able to be with her up until the last 8 hours. It was an incredible experience, difficult but full and rich.

There were moments of great grace and beauty. At one point she was resting, and I pulled out her hymnbook and began to sing to her, songs of crossing over, old favorites. I had a moment where I froze, wondering if I was doing the right thing, if maybe my singing would bother her. But then I flashed on your picture of the music therapist singing to a dying woman that you showed me five years ago and I knew it was all right.

It was your art that gave me the OK to do something that was meaningful for me and, I hope and believe, meaningful for my mother. I think of that photo often and get choked up whenever I describe it to people. But surely there can be no greater measure of a work of art than its ability to comfort and give courage in difficult situations.

Thank you.
Wendy

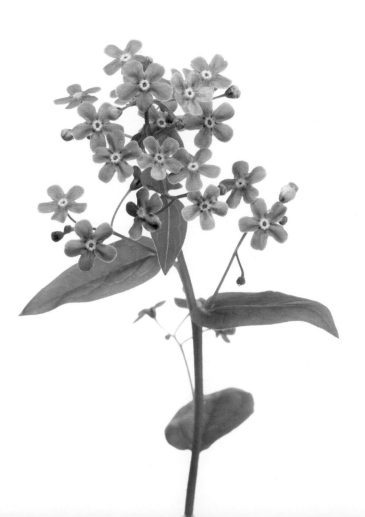

CHAPTER 7

MUSIC AND MEMORY

Because music is processed in many areas of the brain, people with Alzheimer's disease are often able to engage meaningfully and successfully with live music, even those who have severe cognitive impairment. An activities director described it as "holding hands without touching." I can easily relate because every time I photograph groups singing songs from my childhood or youth, I find myself singing along, sometimes with gusto! As Richard Taylor says:

Singing something—anything from children's songs to hymns from the Hallelujah Chorus (I can still recall the first note for tenors) to any and all Beatles songs—helps me feel that I am feeling okay and, in fact, good.

Readers who know my book *Alive with Alzheimer's* will remember Heather Davidson as the music therapist whose magical talents were described throughout an entire chapter. Heather now lives and works near Washington, DC, and I see her regularly for pleasure and for the insight she offers, as below:

The beauty of music is that it does not require one to communicate verbally. Engaging in music together can provide a nonverbal, yet meaningful and in-the-moment connection for the person with dementia and her loved ones, thus bypassing the often frustrating results of verbal exchanges. People with dementia are able to communicate fully with the group and other individuals, using only their voices or instruments. This allows people of all functioning levels to participate in a successful musical experience together without anyone being left out because of lack of verbal ability.

During my work in residential dementia care, I have witnessed people with considerable short-term memory loss claim a particular instrument from week to week, becoming upset if that instrument is given to another member. I have also worked with people who, for example, cannot remember how to get from their room to the dining room, but recall when and where the music therapy group will take place every week. One gentleman used to come every week for the group, one hour early, and wait for me to arrive with "his" drum. Somehow the experience of drumming had moved from short-term memory into long-term memory.

Participating in live music with a group requires us to be present or in the moment, and many people with more advanced dementia live only in this present moment. They often experience memories as if they were the present, talking about past people and events as if they were currently happening. The power of music is never more evident than when you witness a person who is unable to hold a conversation sing all of the words and melodies to the songs of early adulthood. This may even inspire a meaningful conversation about treasured memories.

By providing music therapy experiences for elders with dementia, I do not purport to cure them of this disease or reverse its effects. Rather, I hope to provide some respite, however brief, from the burdens that can weigh heavily on those with dementia and their loved ones. I hope to facilitate present moments of joy, because in health or disease the present moment is really all we have.

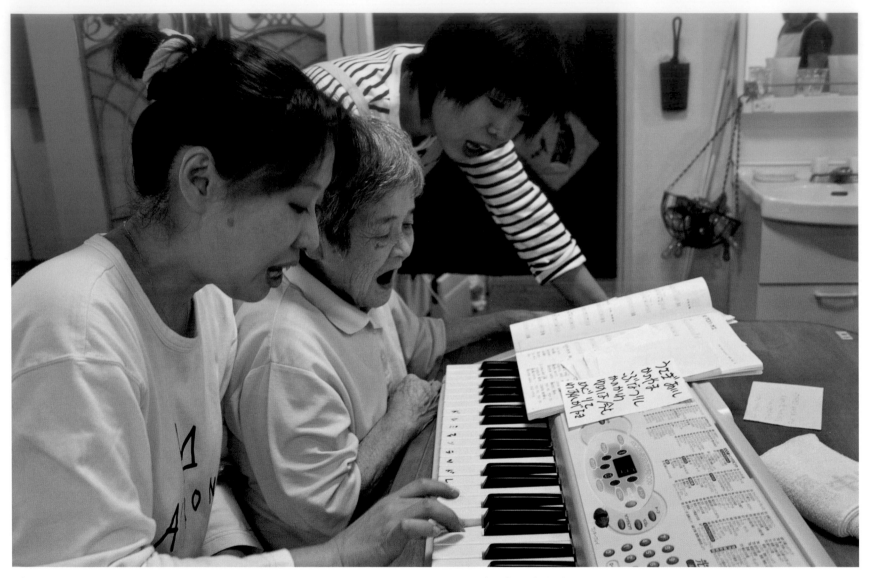

The music group in a Kyoto group home – Japan

The Casio, a portable instrument, was kept in the lounge of this group home. The resident in the photo was trying to play a tune without success. The two staff members listened to the melody she was humming, then began to play and sing it. Together the three recalled the words and they wrote them out so she could sing along.

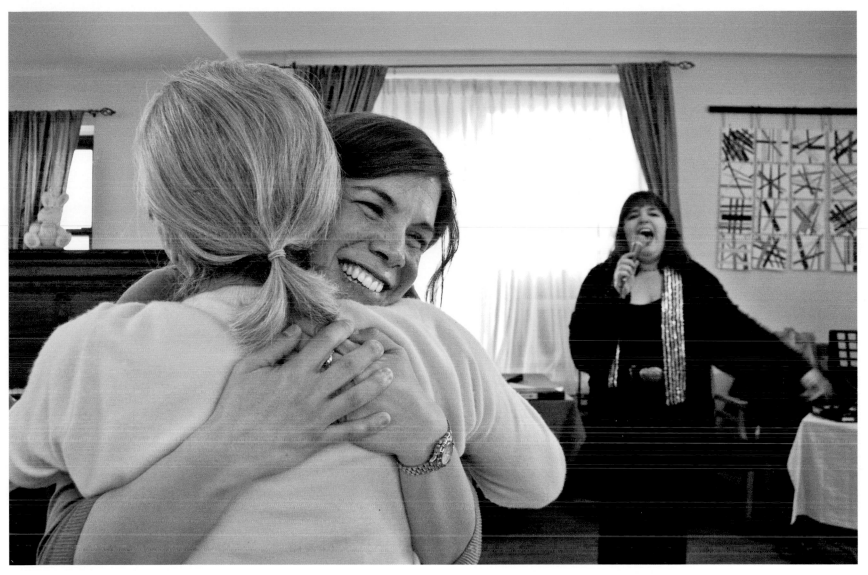

Kerry dancing with Bridget at the Passover party – USA
Linda's entertainment engaged many of the residents at Hearthstone. At first they hummed along, then they began to sing along, and finally, encouraged by Kerry, many of them got up to dance—alone, in pairs, or in groups. In some day programs and residential communities, people with dementia perform in glee clubs and choirs on holidays and at special events.

Music and song are keys to parts of the brain often untouched by Alzheimer's disease. Music and song unlock lyrics, melodies, movement, dance, and every emotion, especially joy. If you do not sing, you are not communicating in a way that touches the soul. A good voice is not required.

—DANIEL KUHN, COMMUNITY EDUCATOR

Mrs. Morimoto sings – Japan

Mrs. Morimoto was the most cheerful resident of a group home I visited in Kyoto. Though she no longer could speak clear sentences, she loved singing. Whenever old songs from her childhood were chosen, she clearly articulated all the words.

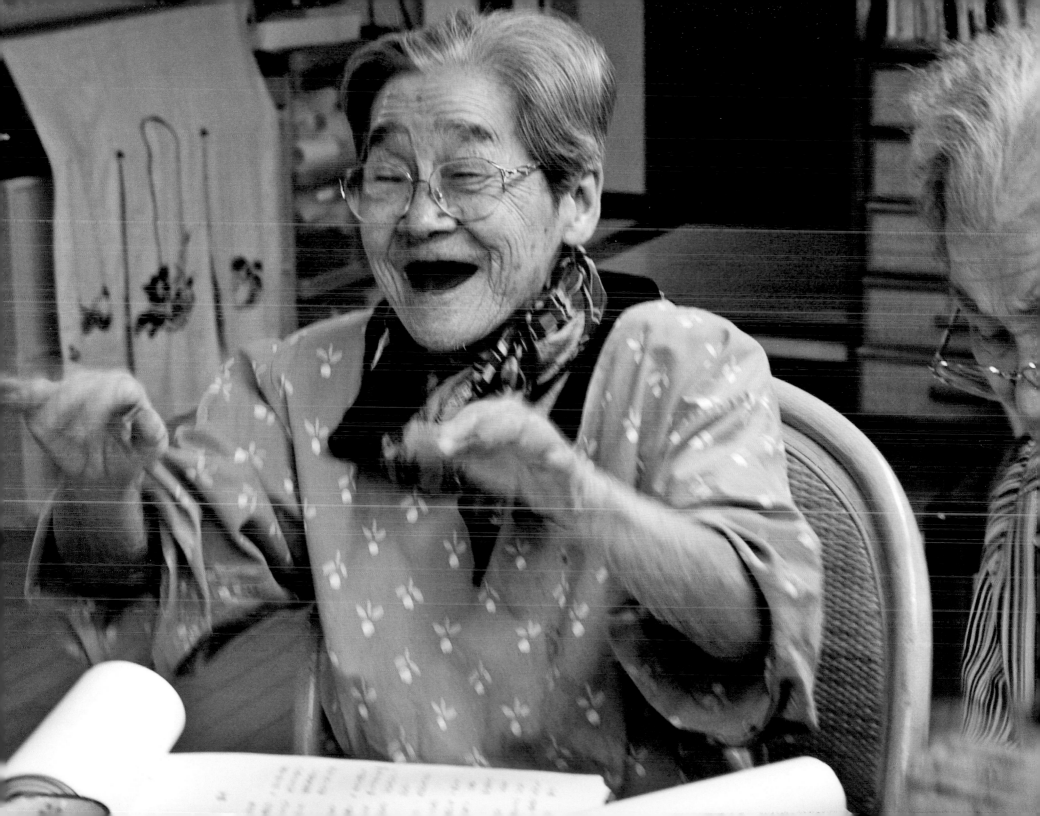

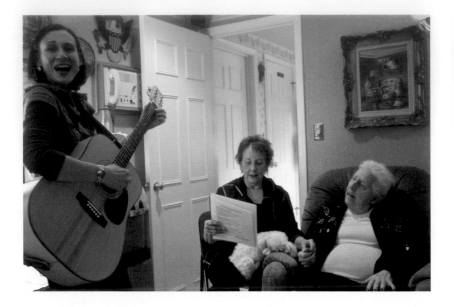 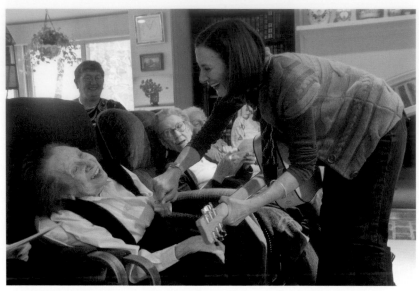

Heather's music therapy at Victoria Home – USA

At Victoria Home, a private, residential dementia community, music therapy is offered twice a week. The first photo here is a three-generation family photo: Helen Jr. is Heather's mother-in-law, and Helen Sr. is her grandmother-in-law. Helen Sr., in addition to being a painter, was a music teacher and amateur pianist and organist. She taught her children and grandchildren to play the piano. During music therapy, Helen Sr. insists on holding a songbook, though she is blind and cannot see the words. Although she now hardly recognizes any of her family members, including Helen Jr., she can sing every song in the book.

The third photo is Heather's favorite. She comments, "Maybe if we all knew that this would be our level of care as we aged, we would not be so fearful of growing old."

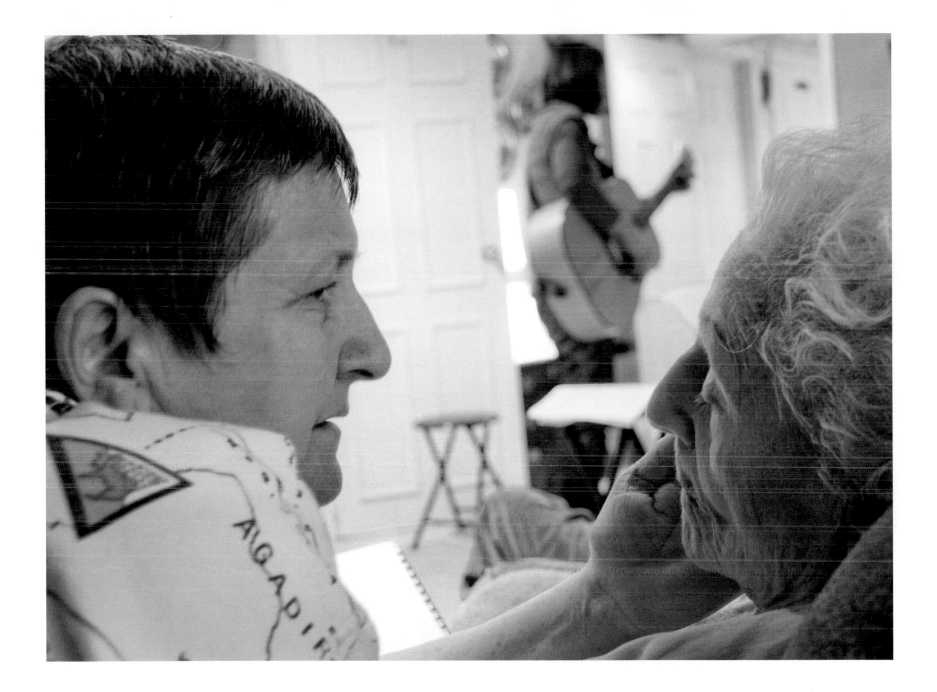

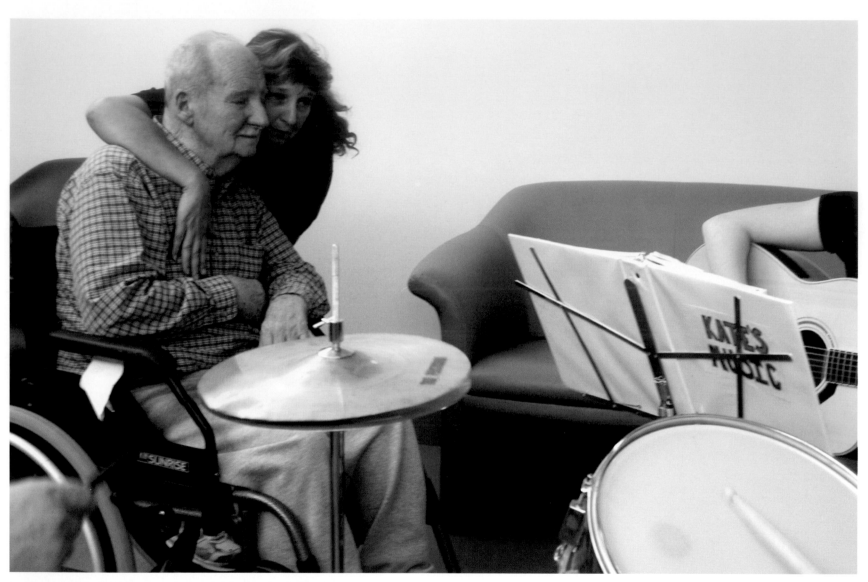

Rollin and his daughter at the Windjammers session – USA

Kate, a music therapist in the Alzheimer's unit of Heather Hill Care Communities, formed a small "band." Three male residents, all with quite advanced dementia, named the group the Windjammers. They loved meeting, jamming, and joking about going "on tour." Rollin didn't want to play this day, but he was engaged with the music, his friends, and his daughter who was visiting. He wept a bit as he recognized a song he knew from his youth, and she wiped away his tears.

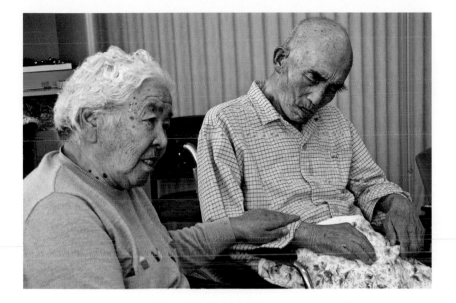

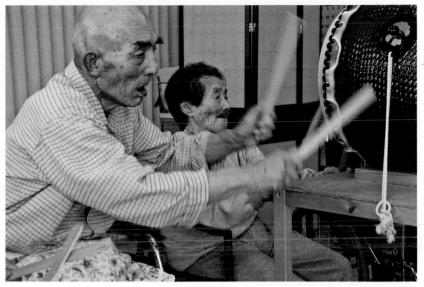

Patient and his wife at a music therapy session – Japan

Despite my strong conviction that music therapy can be effective with almost all people with Alzheimer's disease, I thought it unlikely that the man who came into this session with his wife would participate in any meaningful way. How wrong I was! The second photo was taken only fifteen minutes later. What a change! How good it is that the music therapist didn't write him off for this activity.

Don't underestimate the dragon that sleeps. Some people say, "Memory is everything." Yet it is possible to live predominantly in the present and even to enjoy it. Many stimulation techniques try to reach that goal. What is important is never to forget what is the real interest of the person. It's also essential to remember that any therapeutic approach starts with knowledge of the person.

—PHILIPPE ROBERT, PSYCHIATRIST

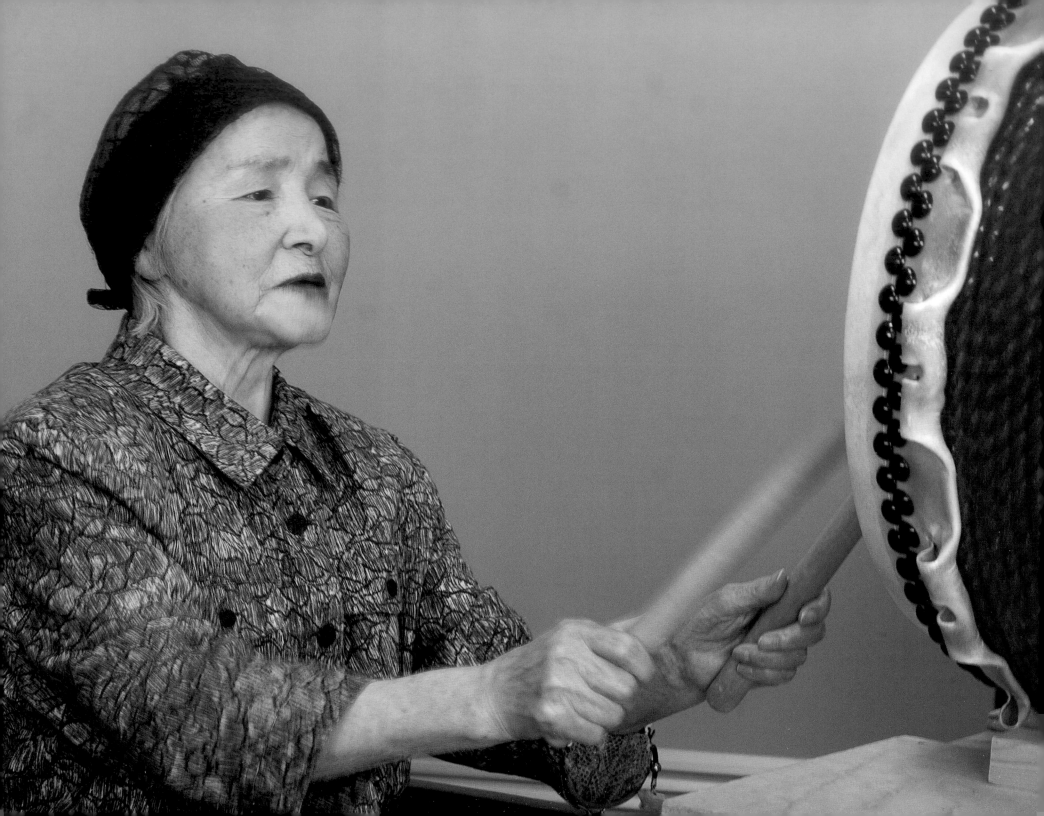

Woman drumming at the Uchida music therapy session – Japan
This lovely woman was in the same drum circle as the man on the previous page. Though she was part of the group, she was caught up in her own intense rhythmic response.

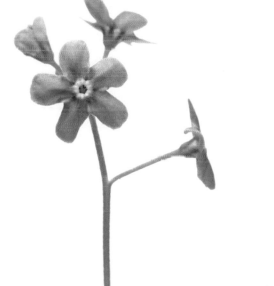

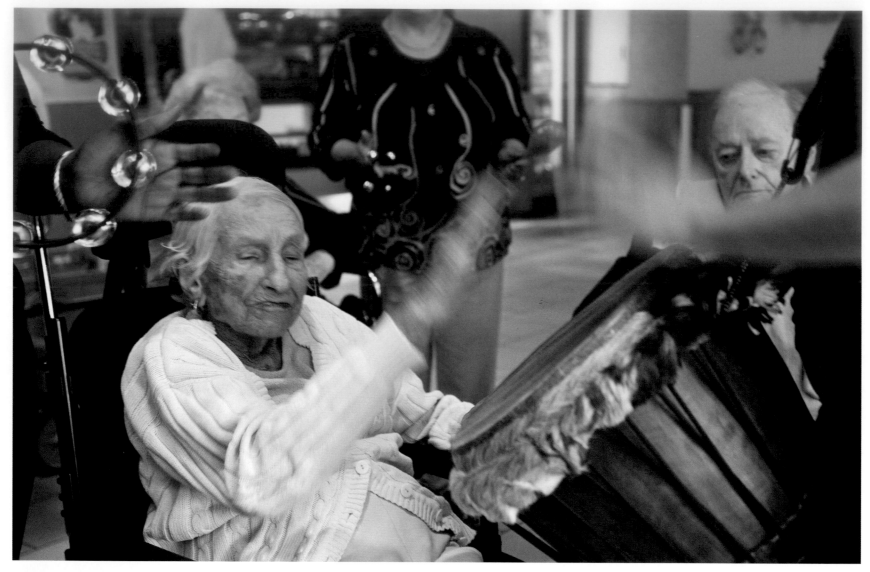

Liliane in the drum circle at Baycrest – Canada
Intense responses to drumming were evident among elderly Jewish residents of
Baycrest in Toronto. Visiting family members and staff joined in as well.

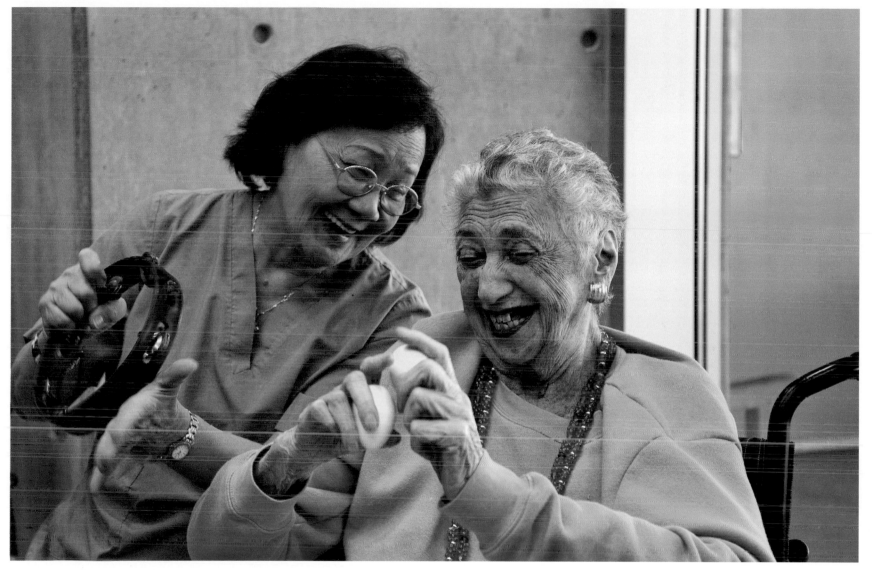

Facunda and Esther at the drum circle at Baycrest – Canada

Facunda and Esther arrived early for the drum circle, knowing from prior experiences that they would love the activity. It was clear to me that in addition to enjoying the music itself, they were happy to have this shared experience.

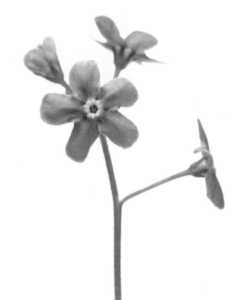

Janette playing the xylophone – USA

Janette, a resident at Heather Hill Care Communities, was on hospice when I met her. A former lawyer, she still had a clear look and a good way of relating to others. Though she was in her last days of life, she was mostly alert and continued to participate in various activities. She particularly enjoyed the music therapy sessions and Reiki massages.

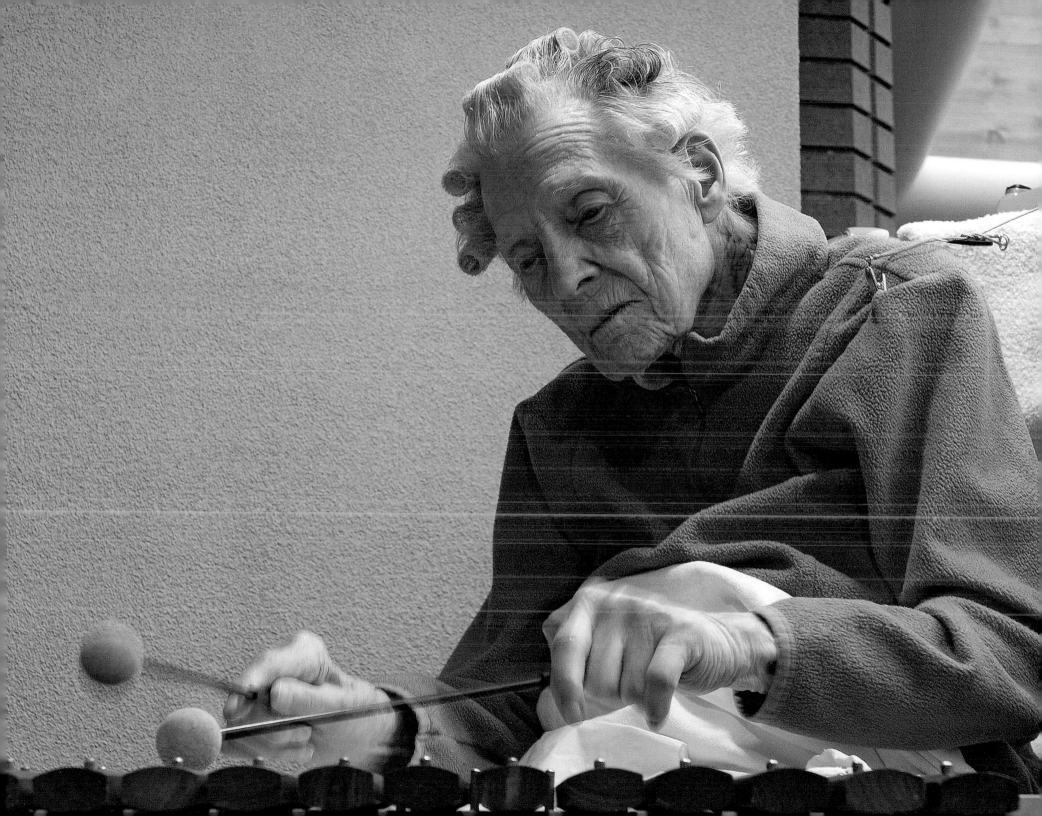

The emotional density seen in a large number of patients with Alzheimer's disease has led many teams to independently develop art therapy programs. Artistic expression through drawing, painting, poetry, music, and dance reveals possibilities for concentration and communication.

In our day-care unit at the Hospital Local in Uzes, France, we made art a priority. We invited painters and musicians from outside the medical world. They captivated our patients, leading them in their procedures, and guiding them into several hours of intense concentration and creativity. We sensed the calm and pleasure in the unit shown by the patients and their relatives during an afternoon of painting, and the euphoria and emotion that reigned during an afternoon of music or dance.

Art can be presented in multiple forms in an institution: through concerts; by producing art; writing or presenting dramatic works; via creating art galleries. These can be offered to patients who are at any stage of the disease.

If the effects art has on symptoms such as depression, speech, communication, and anxiety are fully recognized, we will not limit this approach to one single therapy. The improvement and well-being patients have experienced through art show that fundamental cultural and relational needs are very often, too often, forgotten.

—FRANÇOISE GUILLO-BEN AROUS, GERIATRICIAN

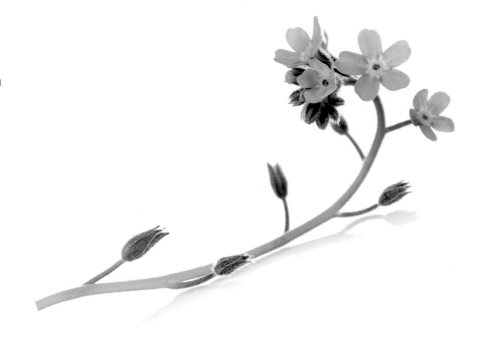

CHAPTER 8

ART AND IMAGINATION

I recently read a headline that said, "Viewing Art Is Like Being in Love." The article referred to research by a professor of neurobiology and neuroesthetics in London, Semir Zeki, who examined the brain activity of people viewing art while inside an MRI scanner. The reward center of the brain, the orbito-frontal cortex, showed increased activity including surges of dopamine, resulting in feelings of intense pleasure similar to the states of love and desire. The study is undoubtedly interesting, but such scientific evidence isn't needed to convince me of the positive effects of art activities for people with dementia. I've often observed them and have heard stories of powerful responses.

Berna Huebner's mother, formerly a painter, had ceased to make art as her dementia progressed. She couldn't speak well, had difficulty connecting with Berna and people at her Alzheimer's residence, and rarely participated in activities. After several refusals, she accepted Berna's encouragement to paint again. Once she began she continued long afterward, explaining, "I remember better when I paint." Berna's film of that title offers a strong vision of the power of art.

Programs for dementia patients that include museum visits are now widespread, and their success has led to visits to films, dance performances, the circus, and botanical gardens. These programs permit engagement with art, connections with other people, and a renewed bond to cultural life. In Chicago a "culture bus" offers people with early stage dementia weekly programs and day trips to cultural sites and events.

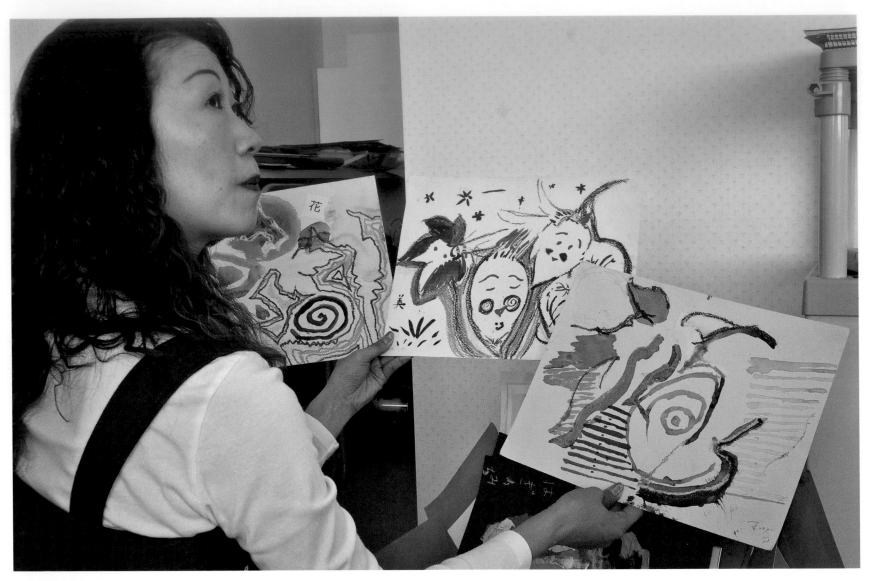

Uchida Hospital art therapist showing patient paintings – Japan
This art therapist kept hundreds of examples of completed, multimedia works done by patients who participated in her program. She was proud of them and their work, and was eager to show me some of their paintings.

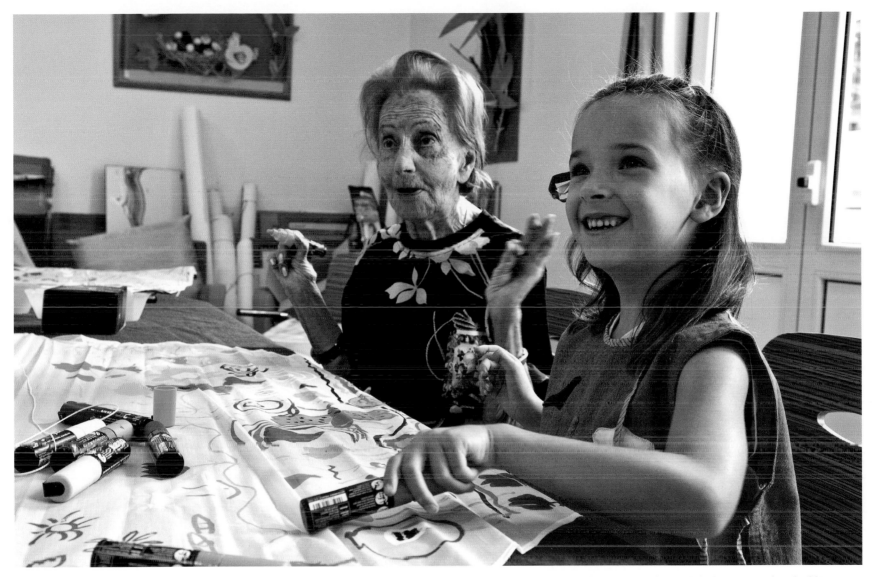

Marie-Thérèse and Féderica painting a kite – Monaco

Despite a ninety-year-plus age difference, Marie-Thérèse and Féderica had a good time painting a kite together. The Speranza Center—Albert II Day Care in Monaco has organized intergenerational paint workshops where children and their older partners are free to express their artistic talents while decorating a hundred kites to be flown in Monaco on September 21, World Alzheimer's Day. The project promotes intergenerational health-care support work and public awareness.

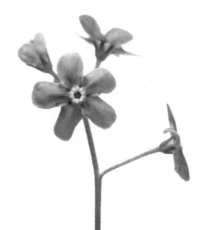

Subbamma engaged in a crafts activity with an aide –India
At the Bangalore Day Care Center, there were a few organized group activities and many individualized ones. Several residents, including Subbamma, enjoy familiar or new art and craft activities.

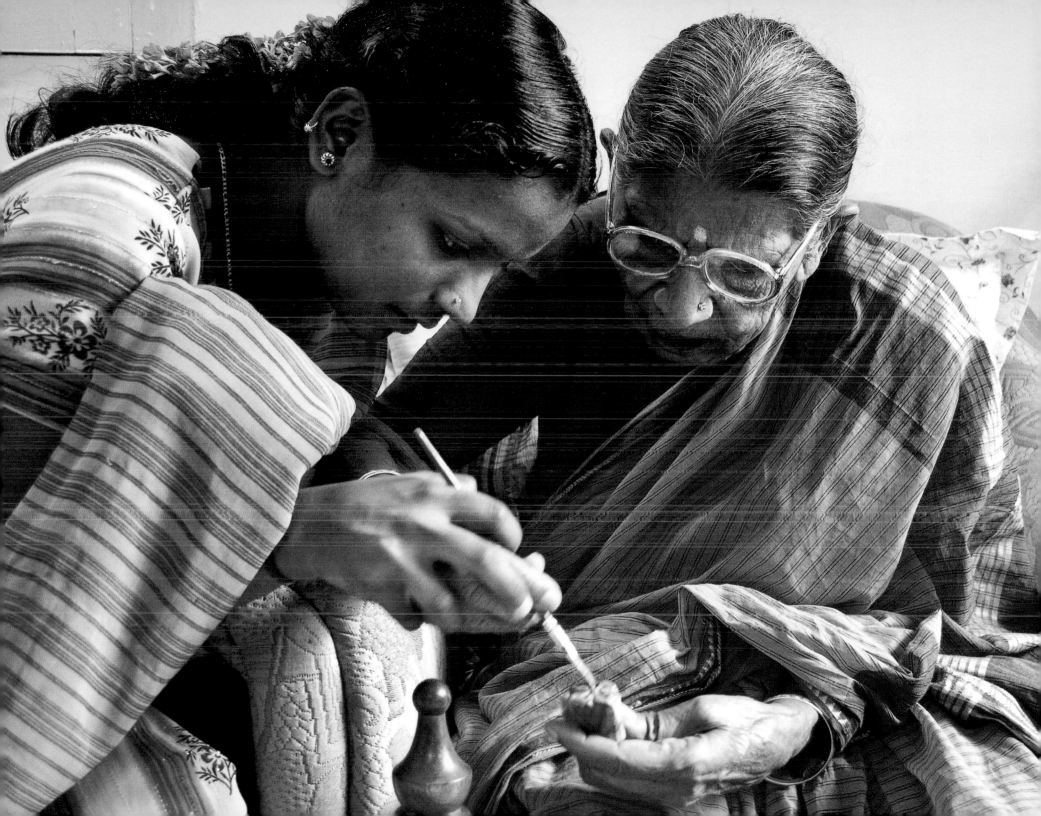

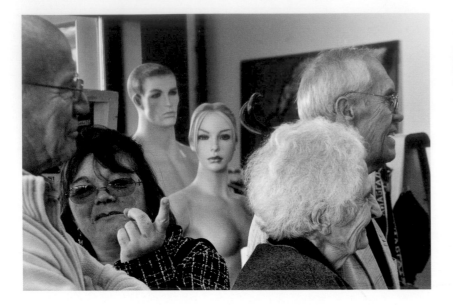 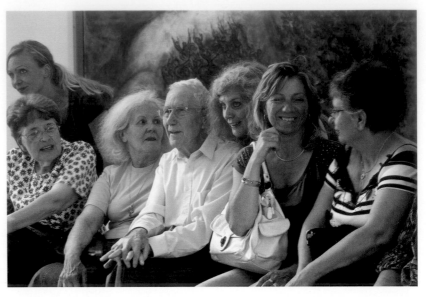

The France Alzheimer plan (2008–2012) promotes
nonpharmaceutical treatments, care for both patients and their
caregivers, and initiatives that help to change the perceptions of the
general public about Alzheimer's and related disorders and about
aging in general. Our collaborative program with the municipality
is targeted not only at creating pleasurable experiences for the
participants, but also at adapting the environment, promoting a
sense of dignity, and encouraging a positive vision of aging. Patients
and their families have been enthusiastic. The program is improving
their integration into their immediate environment: their city.

—VALERIE LAFONT, SPEECH THERAPIST

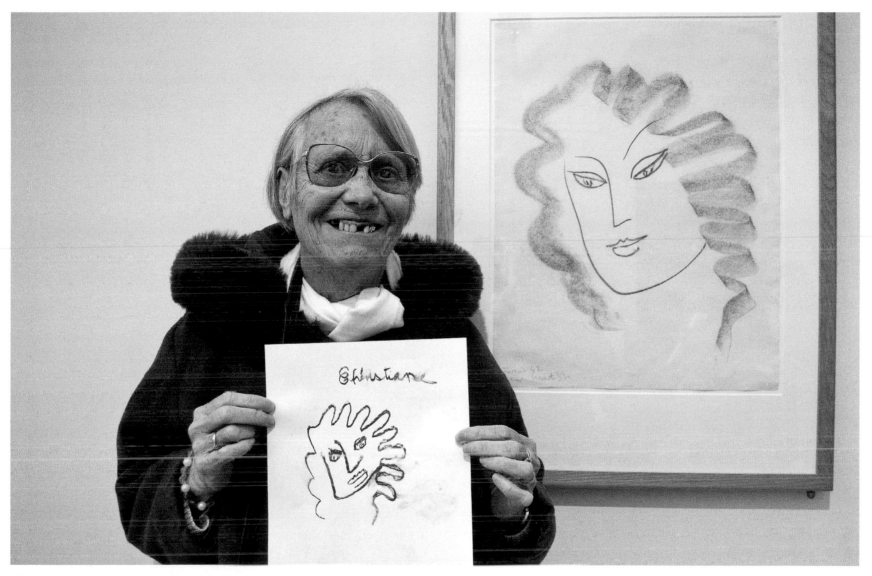

Christiane is proud of her sketch – France

As the last step of a visit to the Matisse Museum in Nice, participants were given sketching materials and invited to try to reproduce the artist's technique. Christiane was very proud of her results, with good reason.

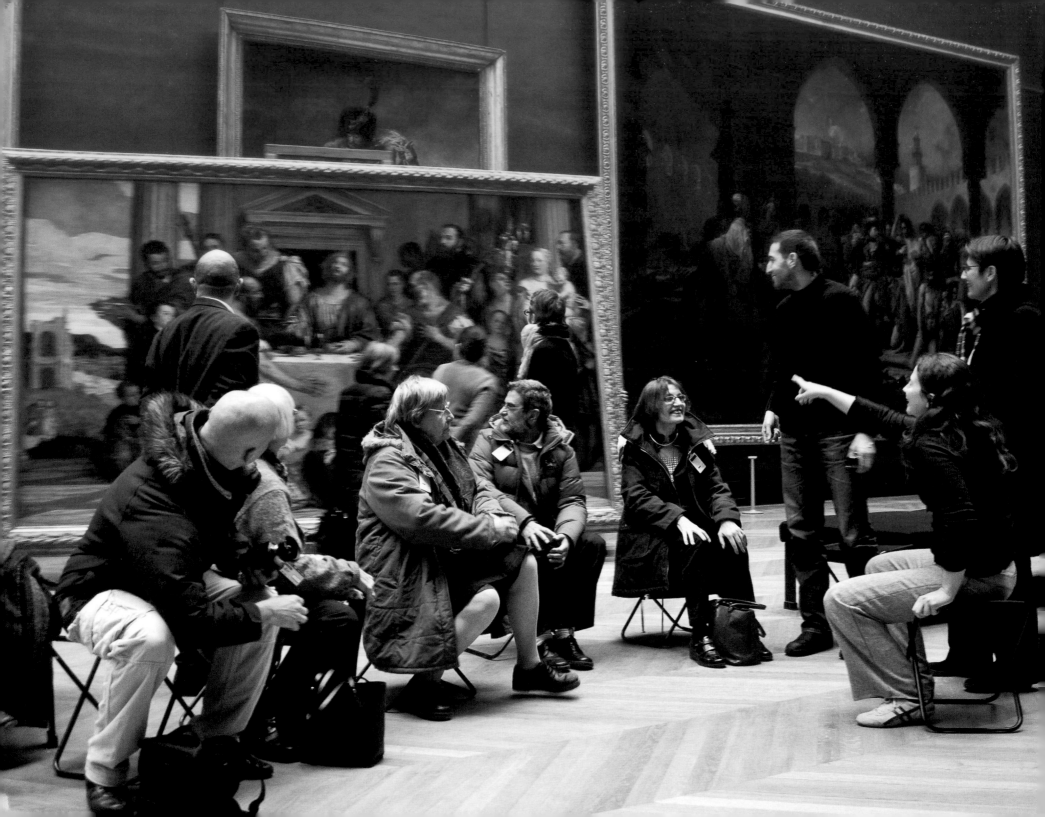

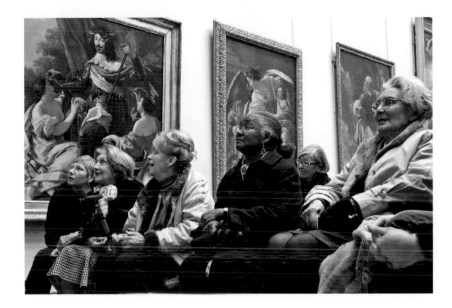

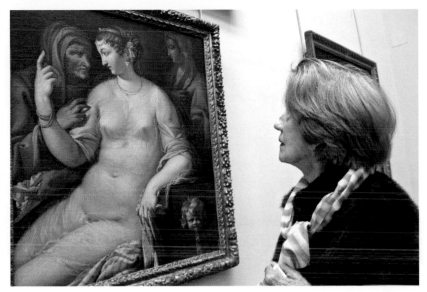

ARTZ visit to the Louvre – France

Cindy Barotte, who has been running the ARTZ program at the Louvre for several years, welcomed me on two visits she organized for people with Alzheimer's. Each participant was accompanied by a volunteer. For two hours the group walked through parts of the museum, talking with one another. They stopped at four or five preselected great paintings where, guided by questions from Cindy, they offered their impressions and interpretations. Occasionally one of the curators added some commentary.

Tuesdays are good days for such visits, as the museum is closed to the public and there is less commotion and crowding. Because it is also a day for staff to clean and do other tasks, there sometimes are surprises. In the photo opposite, a large painting was suddenly being moved through the room we were in.

At the present time, despite the large amount of media attention devoted to them, people with Alzheimer's are frightening to others. This fear results in social exclusion, which in turn reinforces the problems that the person suffers from. In addition, disorientation and weakening relational capacities make it difficult to find satisfying activities outside the home. These deficits lead to a progressive reduction in activities, while the characteristics of the illness and perceptions about Alzheimer's increase affective and social isolation.

The association ARTZ, Artists for Alzheimer's, strives to make cultural places accessible to all, assisting to open them to people with Alzheimer's disease, to bring them pleasure, and to return them to the heart of the society.

—CINDY BAROTTE, EDUCATOR

Much of medicine is palliative. We only cure people sometimes, and in the end the battle to cure is lost. Or is it? The hope of palliative care is, perhaps, that some sort of cure is always possible. The battle against the biology of aging is ultimately lost. But the war, in biological terms, is also about pain, falling, eating, drinking, being sick, losing energy—and something can always be done in these areas to help.

Then there are the psychosocial fields and the spiritual terrain. Here palliative care offers the hope, not of loud victories, but of quiet peace, where the right approach can win hearts and minds. This is why the palliative-care approach is so important for people with dementia. It should instill hope: hope that something can be done, sometimes using medication, but always using psychological understanding. Attention should always be given to the social environment as well as to the physical settings of care, along with an openness to the person's spiritual needs and those of his or her family.

—JULIAN HUGHES, PSYCHIATRIST

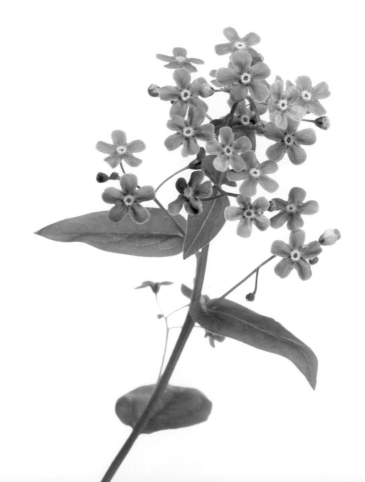

CHAPTER 9

OFFERING CONSOLATION AND COMFORT

Those who deliver person-centered care until the end of life give meaning to Hippocrates's statement, "The art of medicine is founded on observation: to cure sometimes, to relieve often, to comfort always." These practices maintain dignity through small attentions and respectful treatment to patients, and provide moral support to family members. There is never "nothing to do" in terms of providing comfort. I titled an exhibit of photographs about end-of-life care *Gardeners of the Heart,* and I believe the phrase is appropriate.

All of us need consolation from time to time. But the need is greater, so much greater, at the end of life, for both patients and those around them. In Santo Domingo, I accompanied Daisy Acosta, a psychiatrist, on a home visit to a patient. Altagracia had been cared for lovingly by her three daughters, Gilda, Macie, and Viviana, for the sixteen years of her dementia. Now the three daughters were gathered at the bedside of their ninety-three-year old mother. It was not clear whether Altagracia recognized Daisy, but the daughters were deeply appreciative of a physician who would come to their home when many would say there was no reason to visit. The daughter of another of Daisy's patients who had passed away several months earlier said with strong emotion, "Dr. Acosta was always there for both of us, from diagnosis to the cemetery."

Like Daisy, Priyamvada Muddapur knows how to "write the last chapter together." During my stay in Bangalore, Priyam was my hostess, my source of information and insight, my guide to the Bangalore Alzheimer's community, and my friend. Knowing how much I loved the photo of Ashwani and Didi, she sent me news of Didi's death a few months later:

Dear Cathy,

On January 17, 2010, Didi decided to leave us. Your star participant of the Bangalore photoshoot is no more. This has been the most painful incident in my career. I myself took a long time to come to terms with this. I was there with her until the last of her rites were completed. I got to bathe her one last time, dress her one last time, kiss her one last time, before I bid farewell to "my daughter"—remember she used to call me "Mamma"! The end was very quiet and peaceful. She passed on in her sleep.

The family also is going through a lot of distress surrounding her loss. They come to the day center and we relive her memories. We all miss Didi very deeply. Many times I go and sit in the chair that she used to sit in all day long, and I try to feel her presence. I have my quiet time there.

I still have the artwork she used to do for her "Mamma" up in my office. Every time I look at it, I remember her. I also look through the photos of her at the day center. There are so many images that bring a smile; there are so many that bring tears. She was so full of life. She was the one who made me understand that there is so much life to live every single day. She is here in her "mamma's" heart forever safe and secure.

—Dr. Priyam

How wonderful it would be if all professional caregivers for people with dementia were like Daisy and Priyam! How can we recruit such people, train them in Alzheimer's care, reward them well for their efforts?

Touch is our most forgotten sense and yet it can say more than words and remind us of our most human moments and ecstasies.

—PETER WHITEHOUSE, NEUROLOGIST

Harmony House care manager reassuring a frightened resident – India

Mr. Nair was a tough lawyer and businessman, but memory loss and serious behavioral problems that began five years earlier caused difficulties. It became impossible for his family members to manage him at home. At the Harmony House Respite Center, he initially had emotional outbursts and would not listen to staff. Now he is very cooperative, but when another resident became threatening, it was Mr. Nair who was frightened. Happily, Mr. Subramanian, the Harmony House care manager who worked for more than twenty years with leprosy patients, is full of compassion. He has gained Mr. Nair's trust and was able to reassure him.

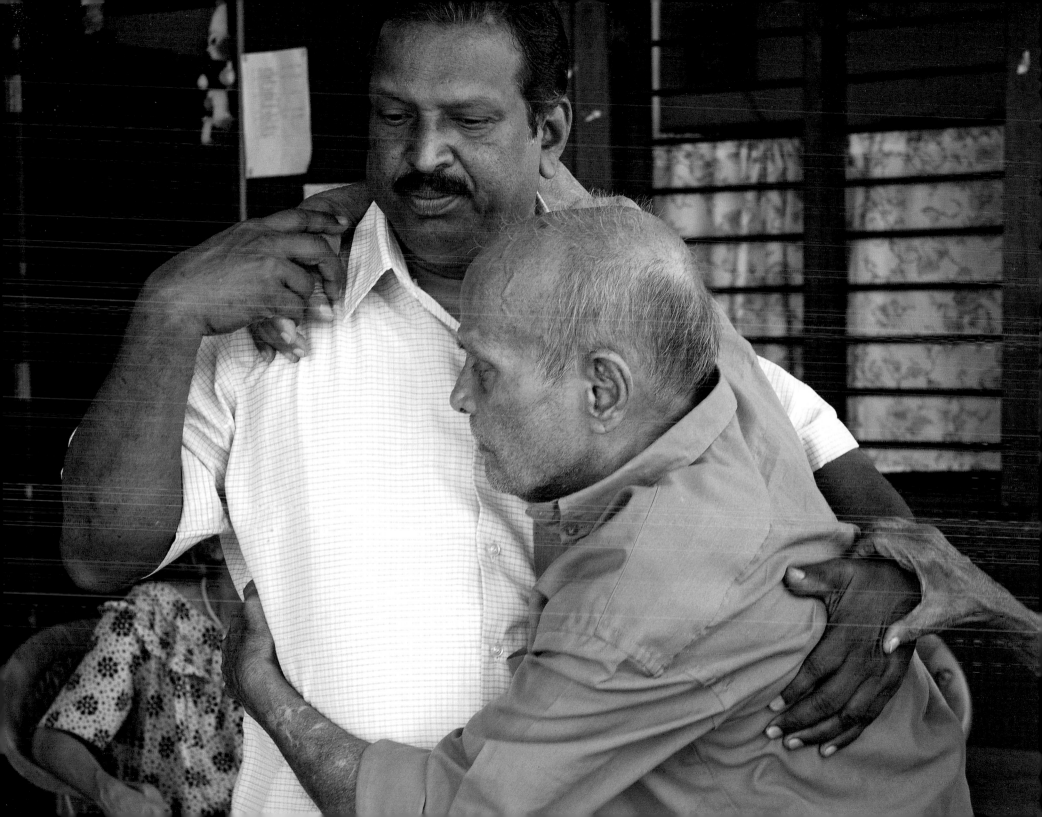

High ideals of volunteerism are an important part of traditional Indian culture. It is not surprising then that promoting meaningful volunteerism has been an important aspect of ARDSI's efforts in each of its fourteen chapters in India. Such efforts begin by identifying and nurturing people who possess key traits, such as a resolve to serve others, a desire to dedicate time proactively, and a willingness to constantly work to increase their knowledge in order to best serve patients and their family members. Strong training programs have been developed to optimize the capacities of those who join. Support mechanisms for volunteers have been ensured. Volunteers help by making regular home visits, operating a dedicated helpline, enhancing the capacities of family members in Alzheimer's care, and enabling access to health- and social-care resources. Where there are day-care programs, they also assist. Volunteers' efforts are regularly recognized through awards in public forums.

—NIRMALA NARULA, ALZHEIMER'S ADVOCATE

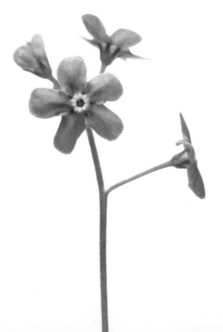

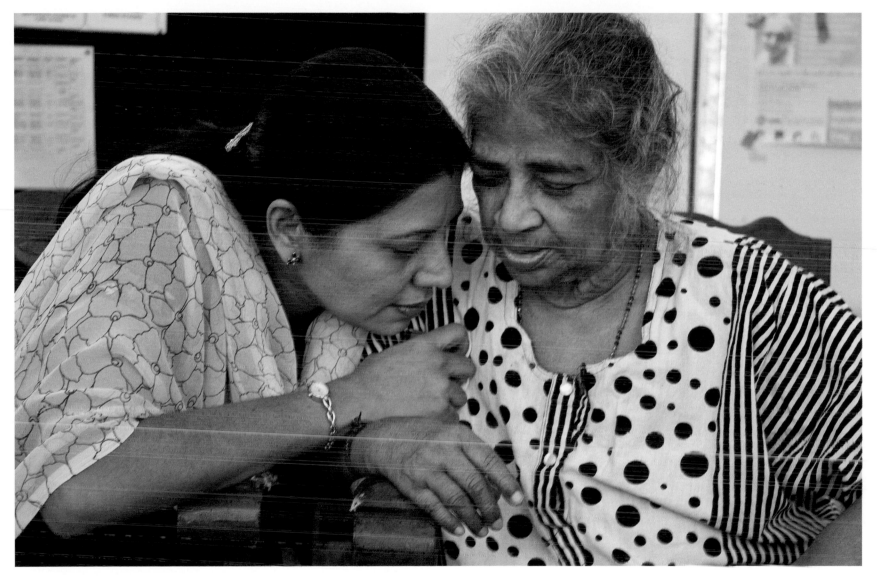

Volunteer consoling a sad woman – India

This participant in the ARDSI day-care center in Cochin, India, was diagnosed with dementia at age sixty-eight and was initially taken care of at home by family and domestic servants. When her aggressive behavior became problematic, she was *enrolled in the day-care center. Here she chats, tells stories, and benefits from trained staff members and understanding and kind volunteers, such as Geetha.*

Ana de Jesus de Bido and her physician husband run a care facility in the Villa Francisca barrio in Santo Domingo. Ana began by giving food to the homeless elderly around her neighborhood. As others heard about it, more and more people came. Ana began to seek support to buy and distribute more food. Today she works in the facility, but continues to make daily rounds in the barrio to feed, to bathe, and mostly to give advice and consultation to needy seniors. This day's round of visits began with Pastor Ana's visit to a woman living with her daughter in a narrow string of rooms. No longer able to walk and having no wheelchair, she is confined to her bed. At the next home, a woman with Parkinson's disease and Alzheimer's lamented her need for dental work as her teeth are becoming very loose. The only regular visitor she had was a niece who recently moved away, leaving her lonely, sad, and often in tears.

Pastor Ana's last visit was with eighty-two-year-old Ana Luisa and her ninety-two-year-old husband Candelario, who has been diagnosed with dementia. Ana Luisa cares for him, cooking and aiding in all ways, but she takes little care of herself, often not eating. Pastor Ana consoled her and explained the importance of caretakers taking care of themselves. Her work is extremely important in the barrio.

—JUANA GUILLERMINA RODRIGUEZ, SOCIAL WORKER

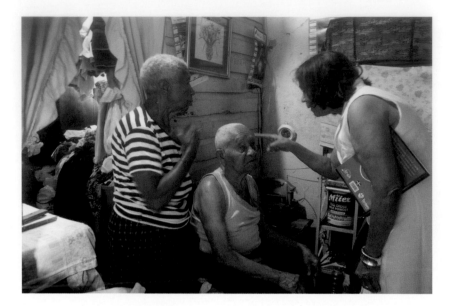

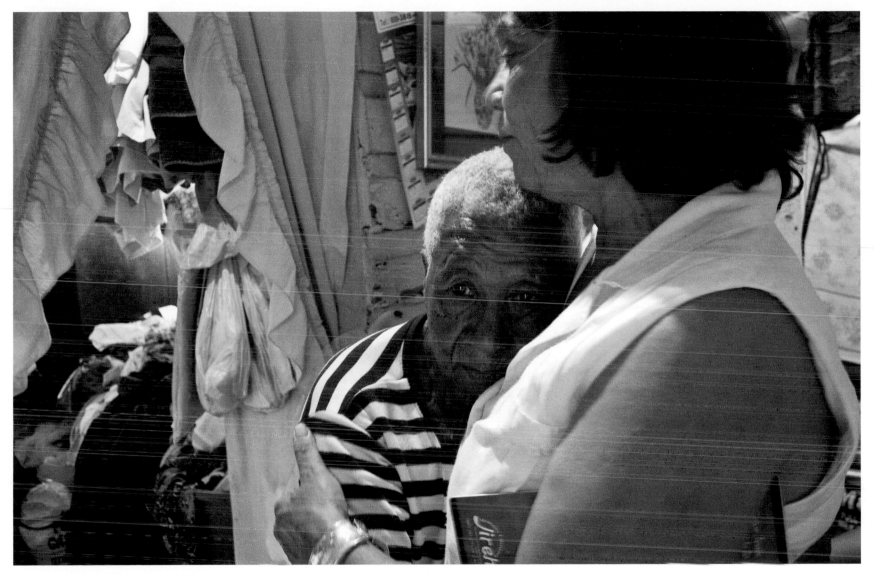

Home visit by a pastor/geriatrician – Dominican Republic
Caregivers for people with dementia need consolation and support, too. Pastor Ana de Jesus de Bido offers this to many of the elderly in the Villa Francisca barrio.

. . . I just long for a face
close to mine, a smile
meant just for me, a silence
I'm invited to share, a chance
To prove there's someone here.

—John Killick, from "Getting Through (1)," Dementia Diary:
Poems and Prose

Alzheimer's makes us different; and "us" refers to all people touched by Alzheimer's—the person, their families, their caregivers. The rules of social engagement change. We let our spouses with Alzheimer's have close relationships with each other and we are happy for it. We enjoy conversations that are animated even though they lack apparent meaning. We ignore that our name is forgotten by our spouse or parent. So what is permissible? That depends. Rules still remain that mandate respect for individual boundaries. A nose rub seems like permissible intimacy to all parties. And how do we get to this new emotional landscape? We see other people acting this way, we follow our hearts, we let go of our old familial roles—and we take on new ones, such as friend.

—JOAN AMATNIEK, NEUROLOGIST

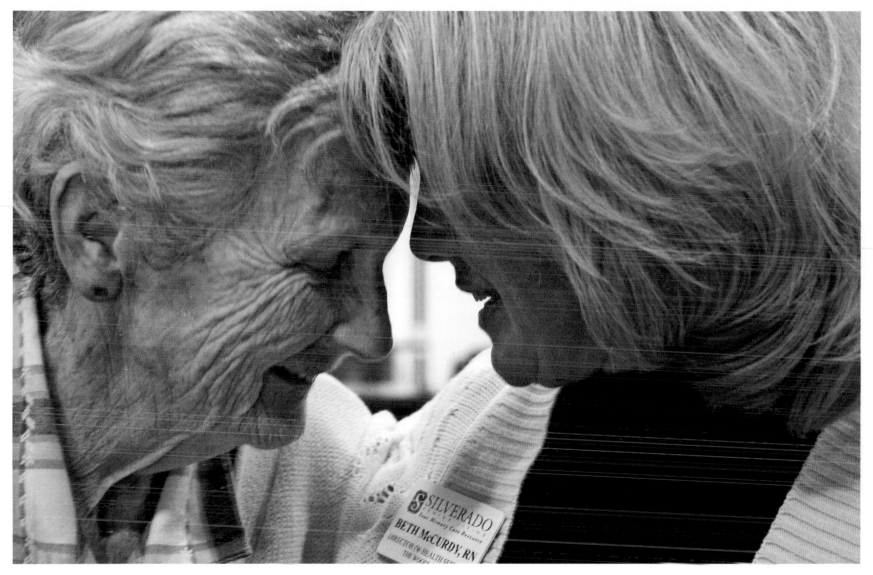

Pat and Beth – USA

Pat had been moving around the care facility with some agitation. Beth's intense focus on her not only created a diversion, but brought her to a totally different emotional state.

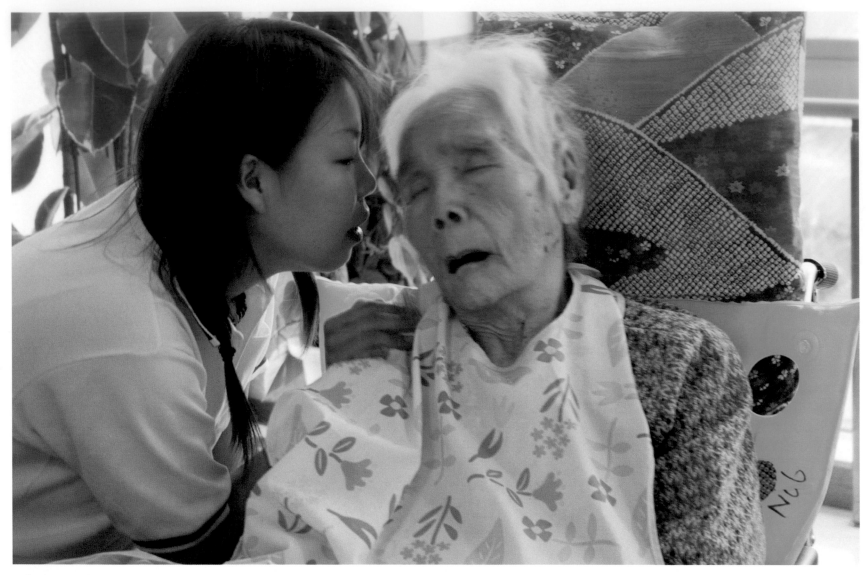

Whisper and a gentle touch – Japan

I have a number of Japanese friends. I learned early that hugs and touching in general were not part of acceptable conduct. Yet when I reviewed the hundreds of photos I took in Kyoto group homes, I was struck by how much physical contact there was

between caregivers and residents. Dr. Yoshio Miyake explains: "In Japan, training courses for professional caregivers of people with dementia take place in many different settings, where nonverbal communication with them including touch or physical contact is emphasized very often."

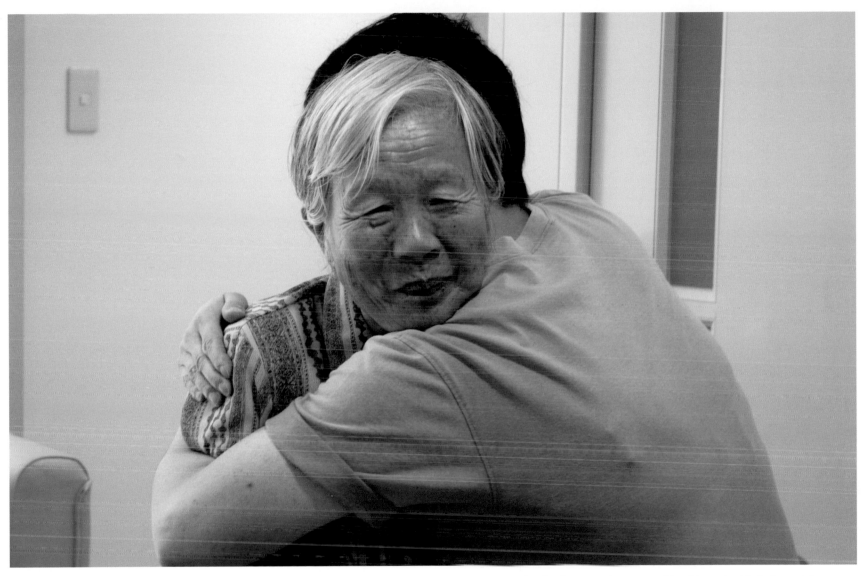

Big hug – Japan

When an aide in a Kyoto group home embraced this resident, everyone smiled. Gerontologist Hidetoshi Endo explains: "Spiritual care at home and in residential facilities is widespread in Japan, offered by care partners with love and smiles. Other recent care practice developments that are considered important include reminiscence therapy, music therapy, and pet therapy, as well as rehabilitation and nutritional support in end-of-life care."

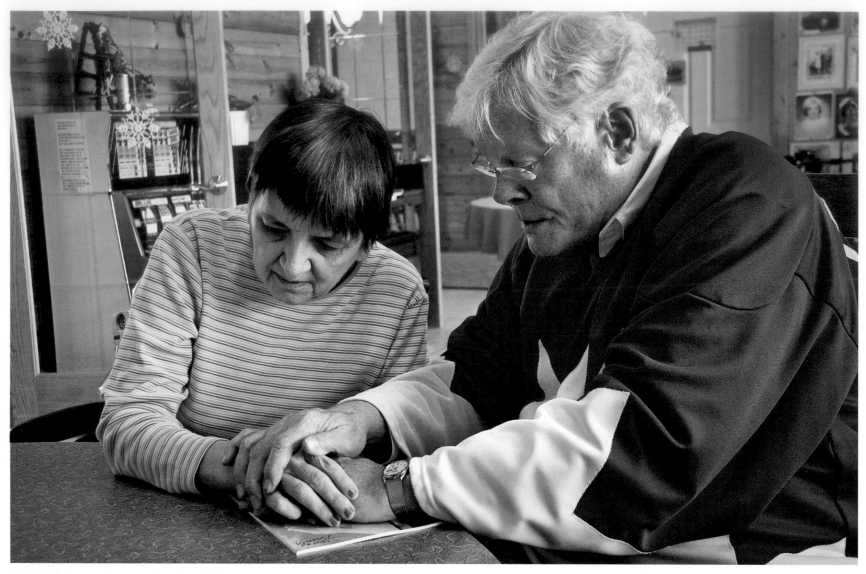

"Everything is going to be all right" – USA

When I began photographing Alzheimer's and end-of-life care, many staff and volunteers told me, "I get more than I give." It took me a while to understand this, but I now know it often is so. Here is an example: I was at Lakeview Ranch with Laurence Harmon, a lawyer and businessman in the Twin Cities. I noticed that he became quite emotional during his interaction with Kay, a sixty-one-year-old patient who had been ill for ten years. He later explained (see text opposite).

Judy Berry, the founder and director of the ranch, told us that although Kay had sometimes been difficult to deal with at home and in other facilities, she has been generally cooperative and happy at the ranch. I watched her interact with Laura with interest. As they were winding up, Judy asked me to give Kay a hug, explaining, "Kay really likes hugs."

Unfortunately, I've had personal-space issues since childhood, and I'm extremely uncomfortable in social situations when I'm expected to hug/kiss or be hugged/kissed by people I don't know, a problem that was compounded for me because Judy had previously warned me about Kay's history of violent behavior.

I gave Kay a halfhearted hug, and sat down with her. She showed me the book she was reading, and we started looking through it together. I was extremely anxious at this point, red-faced for sure, and perspiring. Maybe five minutes into it, Kay reached over to me and held my little finger, which really startled me, but I reached over and covered her hand with mine. She reciprocated; I reciprocated, too.

Then she leaned over to me and said, "Everything is going to be all right." She whispered it again, twice. We just sat there like that for several minutes, and I calmed down immediately.

Afterward, I asked Judy what she and her staff would say to soothe Kay when she would become agitated. You guessed it: "Everything is going to be all right." Kay, end-stage, had used her own calming phrase to comfort me! It was an astonishing, amazing experience for me.

—LAURENCE HARMON, LAWYER

Isn't it wonderful how much intuition Alzheimer's patients have . . . they seem to look deep into our hearts!

—CLAUDIA BAYER-FELDMANN, PSYCHOLOGIST

In 2009 Dr. Françoise Guillo-Ben Arous showed me a Snoezelen room at a hospital where she had created an Alzheimer's program in southern France. No patients were being treated, so I saw only the large room with its lighting effects, music, scents, a water bed, areas to provide tactile experiences, and large tubular water-filled columns with bubbles and colored lights. The concept, she explained, was that the delivery of stimuli to many senses could assist in calming agitated people. The lighting, atmosphere, and process can be changed depending on the needs of the particular person.

Most of the thousands of Snoezelen rooms now in existence are used for therapeutic interventions for people with autism, but they have been found to be effective with dementia as well. I was intrigued, but without seeing how a therapist worked in such a space I was still mystified. Françoise explained the principles to me:

In cases of extreme illness, patients are often best assisted by care that entails mothering behaviors and caresses, strong commitment, and close physical proximity to them. Whether spontaneous or planned, such attentions embody the original essence of caring. The energy of the relationship is concentrated during these times where the caregiver meets the patient fully.

The desired state of calm, of openness, of relaxation is very difficult to achieve in some patients, but it occurs more naturally in the fetal environment of the Snoezelen room, where light, water, twilight, and smells promote the reduction of the patient's resistance. The Snoezelen room, developed and produced in the Netherlands based on scientific medical understandings, helps the therapist to offer the maternal model of care as the paradigm of relationship care. It offers a place for relaxation away from the pressures of a group.

The Snoezelen room allows patients suffering from Alzheimer's disease to reduce or relieve symptoms such as agitation, anxiety, depression, wandering, sundowning syndromes, and to improve mood. It is a noninvasive and relational approach to helping patients and family feel happier.

More than a year later, Bénédicte Cossève, a psychometrician, offered me the opportunity to observe and to photograph while she worked with three people in the Snoezelen room at the Villa Helios in Nice. It was an extraordinary experience watching her skilled and beautiful motions and expressions, which brought about impressive transitions in the patients. Afterward, Bénédicte described what transpired in the three forty-five-minute sessions with Marcel, Jacqueline, and Roseline.

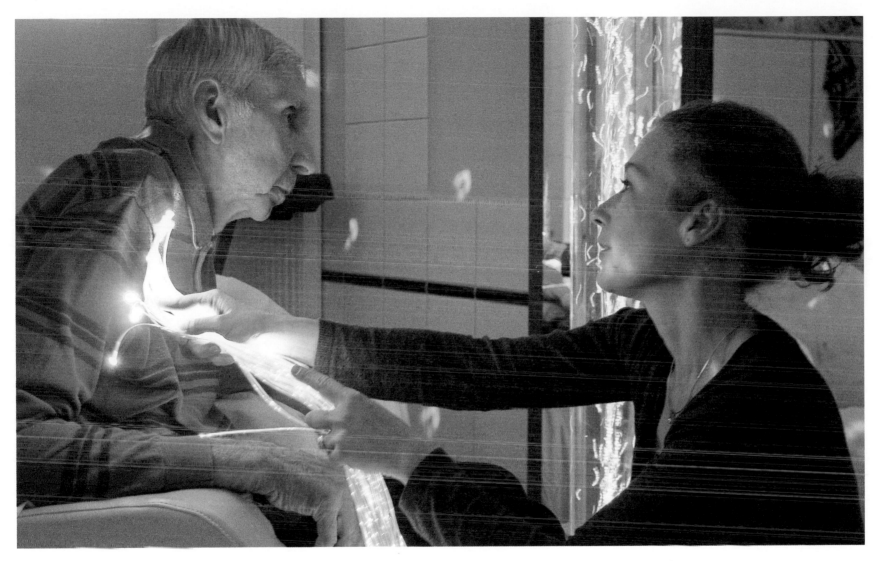

Marcel and Bénédicte – France

"Marcel accepted my invitation to explore the Snoezelen space, and he was quickly attracted by the column of bubbling liquid. The rocking chair that moves slowly according to a rhythm he establishes allowed Marcel to concentrate, and above all to accept my presence. Even better, although he avoided exchanging glances with me, he showed that a relationship was possible by discreetly putting his hand on mine. Thus, it became an exchange between equals, minimizing the professional–patient distance. Through this time together, Marcel, a man who frequently walks around threatening others, became tender, available, and protective. He became another man, or rather, finally became himself." —Bénédicte Cossève

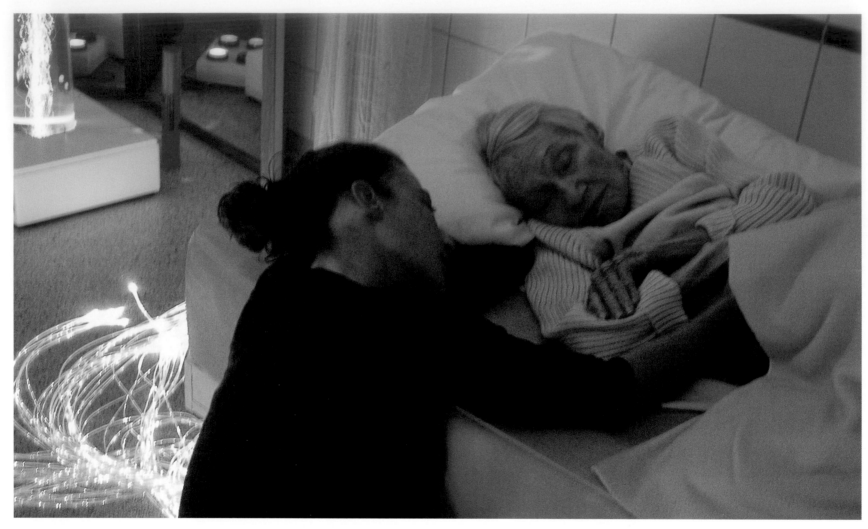

Jacqueline and Bénédicte – France

"Jacqueline cannot sit up without supports anymore, and does not walk, so I lifted her from the wheelchair onto a heated water bed, wrapping her well in a soft blanket. The ambience in which she was bathed is created by a dimly colored light, essential oils, but also my multisensorial presence. At first I lay next to her so she could feel my breath, listen to my humming, feel my respectful touch that gives her security and allows her to experience my adaptation to her rhythm. In a new position, she also could see a loving look. Over the course of the session, Jacqueline, who had arrived in a closed, contracted, painful posture that limited any possibility of exchange, was transformed. Her body opened, her face relaxed, her hands unclenched. Finally we looked at each other with wide-open eyes, sharing the pleasure of the meeting and the moment of well-being."
—Bénédicte Cossève

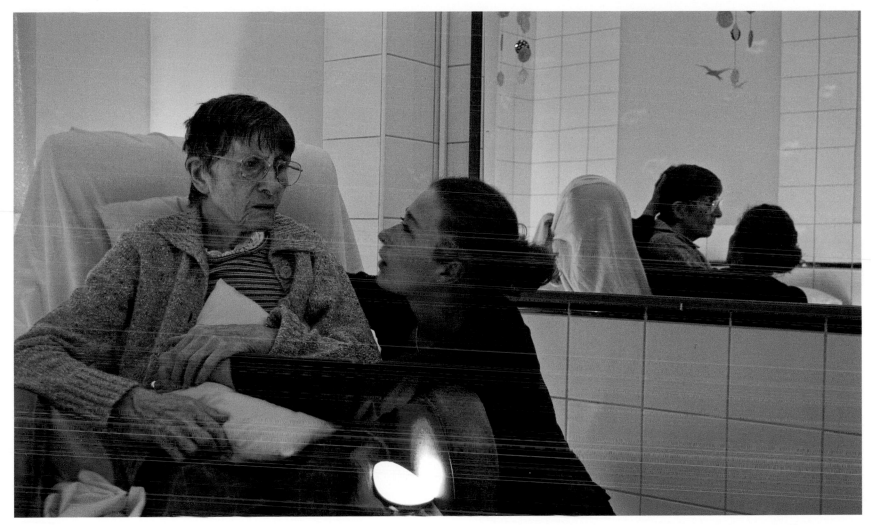

Roseline and Bénédicte – France

"Roseline is said to have no memory left, but she spontaneously sits in the same armchair each time she comes to the Snoezelen. Looking at the changing colors of the room, listening to relaxing music in the background, holding a reassuring cushion pressed against her stomach, Roseline was beginning to enjoy a moment of rest from her permanent agitation and anxiety. I sat near her, making my presence known by voice and by touch, thus inducing relaxation through breathing patterns.

Roseline began with persistent lamenting about her fear and her head- and stomachaches, laments she makes regularly in the other program areas. Soon she fell asleep for a brief instant, serene and relaxed. When she awakened she said spontaneously, "This is really helping," and even inquired about my well-being. The session ended with reciprocal thanks. This turned out to be one of Roseline's last moments of relaxation and sharing as she passed away a few days later."
—Bénédicte Cossève

Palliative care is person-centered care. To be a person is many things. Palliative care recognizes this and takes as its premise the need to look after the whole person. Holism is about seeing people broadly—seeing them in a context of family, place, society, culture, and history. But this is not to lose sight of the person in the center, who will continue to have physical and psychological needs. This person's spiritual needs may be met by the brahmin, the imam, the priest, the rabbi, or some other religious leader. But they may also be met by using personal meditation or complementary approaches to health care involving touch, smells (for instance, aromatherapy), music, or the simple contemplation of nature and enjoyment of open spaces. Spiritual peace also comes from being together with others. But the vista that opens up for people in the context of palliative, holistic care is quite different from the reality of so many "homes" for people with dementia. We need vistas of hope.

Palliative care also involves many ethical decisions. Part of the context here is that life is ending. We need to maintain quality of life—through music, interaction, gentle touch, carefulness, and sensitivity—to the end. But decisions for, with, and about the person must be made in the knowledge that life is coming to an end. In these circumstances, not to accept the concrete reality of the closeness of death would be unwise. Instead, a palliative approach will aim to keep the person comfortable and always to treat the person as valued, but will accept that aiming at cure will not always be appropriate. A peaceful death, which may require the full armamentarium of biological, psychological, social, and spiritual approaches, is the aim and will allow a sense of reconciliation, perhaps, to those left behind. Palliative care is also about grieving and the bereaved. In the end, palliative care is not just about dying well, it is about living well, too.

—JULIAN HUGHES, PSYCHIATRIST

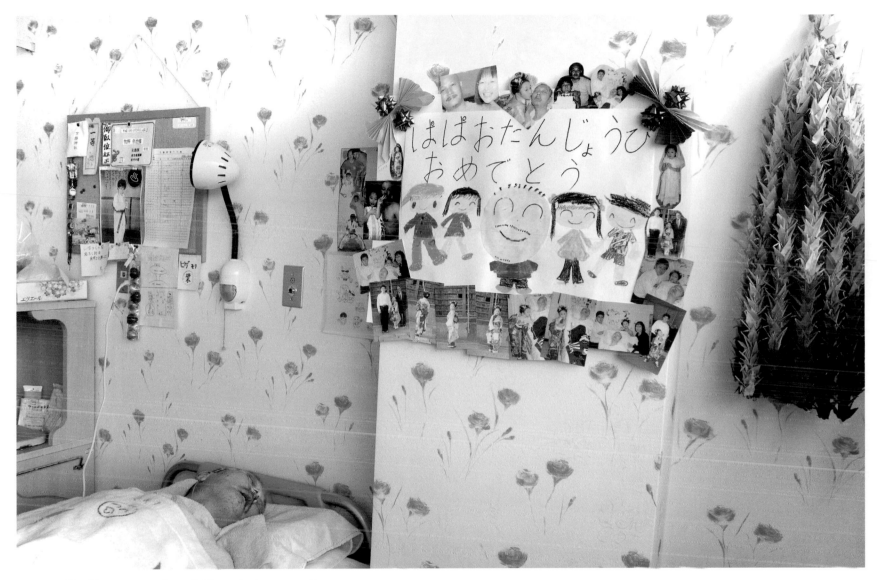

Terminally ill man in a cheerful hospital room – Japan

The delicate flowered wallpaper in this man's hospital room is intended to create a warm and homey environment. A child's drawing is surrounded by photos, a number of which were taken here.

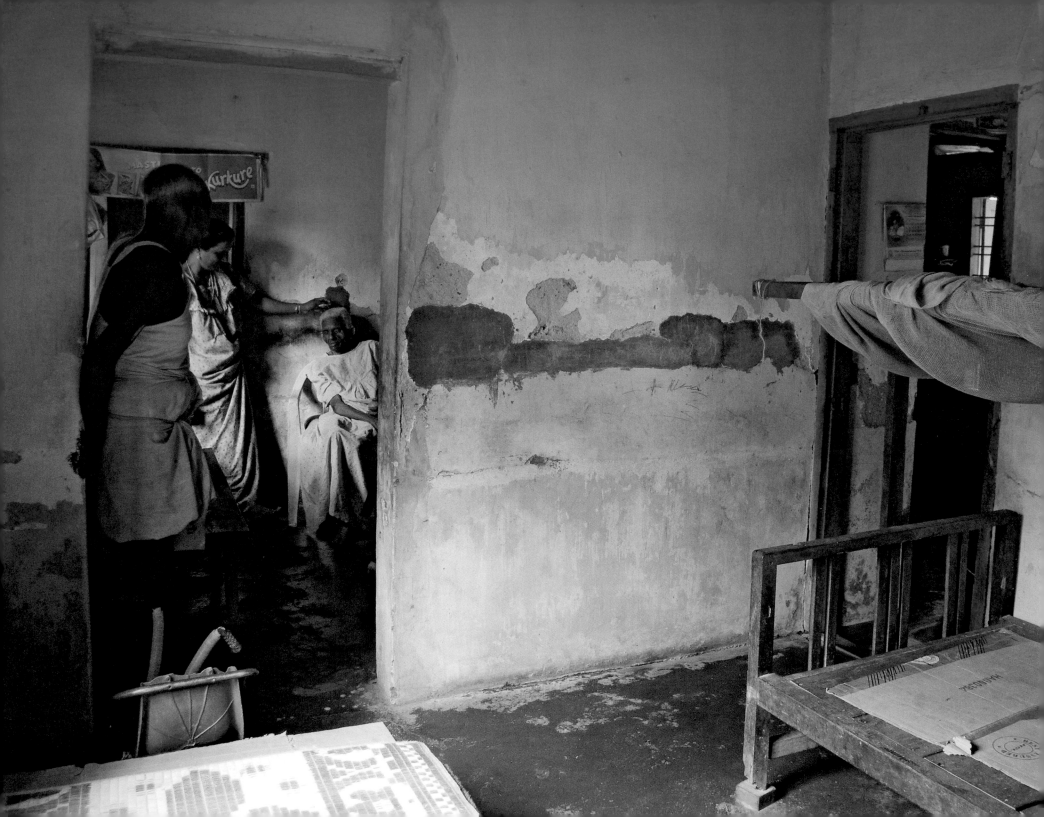

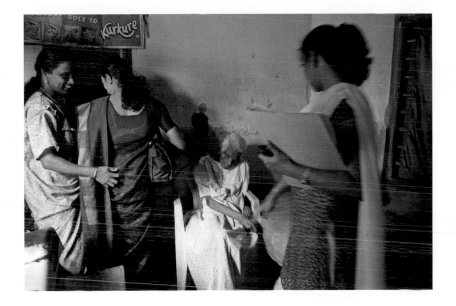

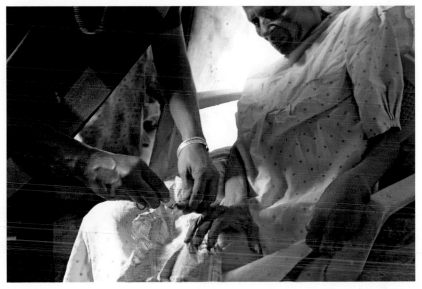

Providing home-based care to people with dementia is an integral part of the comprehensive care program by ARDSI's Cochin chapter. After initial screening, those suspected to have dementia are seen by a psychiatrist and social worker to confirm the diagnosis. Once it has been confirmed, a plan for providing home-based care is created, based on the needs of each individual family. Home care includes giving the right information, offering tips on care, and providing medical and nursing care the patient needs. The most demanding situations are those patients who are bedridden and incontinent.

ARDSI provides this service to the poor and to people in middle-class families rather than to the very rich. Now the project is being expanded to cover people from all social and economic classes with the support of the government.

— K. JACOB ROY, PHYSICIAN AND FOUNDER OF ARDSI

Home visit to the woman in the turquoise room – India

In India abject poverty does not prevent continuing care for people too weak to go out for medical and other attention. Clipping nails, giving a massage, and offering other small attentions are some of the things done by a nurse and social worker at this and other homes in Cochin. They are well received by family members, for whom moral support and little attentions to their loved one are of great importance.

. . . You seem already almost through
the door that opens for us all,
but cannot tell me anything
of what lies on the other side.
Closer, yet further away?

Your body speaks the lines
your mouth can no longer utter
and I am here to learn them.

Each posture, every gesture,
that glint in the eye, cry, turn down
of the mouth, pressure of the fingertips—

are not to be taken in isolation,
but make up a composite
of who you were and are.

So, before it's too late, may I
be your ghost-writer? Let's create
this last chapter together.

—John Killick, *excerpt from "Getting Through,"* Dementia Diary:
Poems and Prose

Quiet end of her journey – USA

I only "met" this patient when she was at the end of her life. The family was visiting, and they were greatly pleased at the gentle care she was receiving at a Silverado community in Texas. Her bed had been turned so she could benefit from the light and warmth. Beth, the head nurse, noted that this resident never wanted to be seen without lipstick, so part of their terminal care was making sure they regularly put lipstick on her.

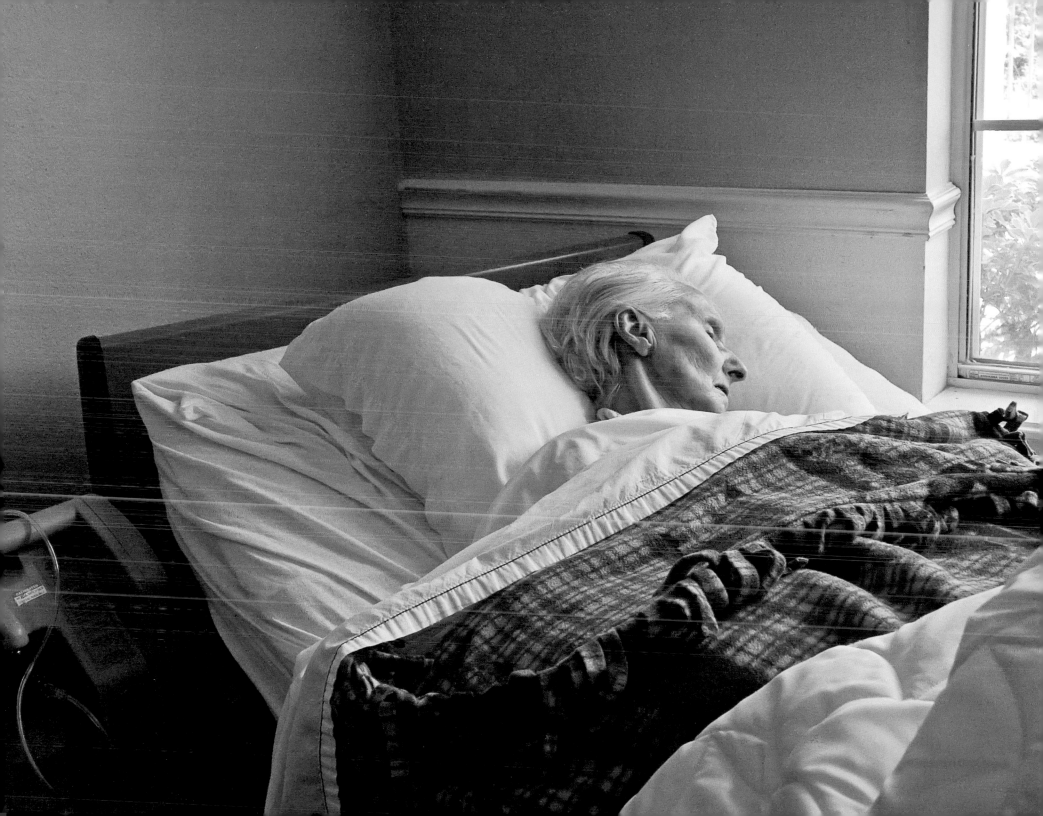

ACKNOWLEDGMENTS

To adequately thank all the people who helped me with this project I would need many pages. The abbreviated statements here are just the tip of the iceberg. I hope that all who contributed recognize the depth of my gratitude.

Kathy Greene, director of the Silverado Senior Living Escondido residential community in 2001, and now a company vice president, was the first person to help me to see Alzheimer's differently when I photographed for *Alive with Alzheimer's*. Kerry Mills, as activities director and then director of Hearthstone residences in New York, brought love and laughter to my mother and the other patients as well as to visiting family members. Dr. Françoise Guillo-Ben Arous, a French geriatrician and close friend, has taught me by words and example about incorporating joy into serious dementia care and into life in general.

As I began to develop a first draft of the photo-driven book, professors Charles Traub and Randy West at the School of Visual Arts, NYC, and Dewi Lewis, president of Dewi Lewis Publications in London, encouraged my creating a trade book. Dr. Joan Amatniek brought her knowledge of journalism, art, dementia, caregiving, and neurology to helping shape the themes of the initial draft. Graphic designers Kiki Bauer and Kevin Greenblat helped turn my rough layout ideas into concrete materials to share with potential publishers. Gil Peytraud worked diligently with me on the preparation of digital files.

Later I was aided in the task of photo editing by the generosity and talents of Jean Caslin and Diane Gregory (Caslin Gregory Associates), Dr. Ferris Olin (Institute for Women and Art, Rutgers University), Pascal Philippe (Courier International), Daphné Anglès (*New York Times,* Paris), Valerie Lafont (CMRR, Hospital Network of Nice) and Diana Edkins (president, Diana Edkins Fine Art Photography Advisory, former director of Exhibitions and Limited-Edition Photographs, Aperture Foundation).

Marc Wortmann, executive director of ADI helped find financial support for the book and related exhibits and obtained the invaluable ADI endorsement. He has been a wonderful partner and a friend. He and Sarah Smith selected sets of my photographs for ADI's publications, generating more widespread interest in the work through the three *World Alzheimer's Reports* (2009, 2010, and 2011) and other materials. Dr. Daisy Acosta, chair of ADI from 2009–2012 and Dr. K. Jacob Roy, chair of ADI for 2012–2015) provided access, hospitality, and encouragement when I photographed in their countries, and friendship since then. Anne Molinier sought me out after seeing an exhibit of my photographs and invited me to work with Nutricia. Steve Graves expanded my connection to this fine company. At Lundbeck, Nuno Ribeiro and Tina Bengtson provided the impetus for the company support of the book.

I am also grateful to those people who invited or curated exhibits of the project photographs: Dr. Judith Salerno and JD Talasek for a six-month exhibit at the National Academies of Science, Washington DC; Dr. K. Jacob Roy for a traveling exhibit around India; Kathryn Kliszat for an exhibit at The LightHouse Gallery, Wolverhampton, UK; Aviva Babins and Bianca Stern for a show at Baycrest, Toronto; Sue Scott, Jane MacFarlane, and Bill Dunne for a show at Glasgow Caledonian University; Lucy Gillan and Juan Tomas for shows at the Fundacion Reina Sofia, Madrid, and in other cities in Spain; Dr. Tarun Dia for an April 2012 exhibit at WHO headquarters in Geneva.

I am indebted to my agents, Karen Gantz Zahler and Judith Ehrlich, whose experience, efforts, and advice helped guide this book to trade publication. Among their contributions was the introduction to Dr. Joyce Starr, whose editorial expertise and coaching skills helped refine the manuscript at several stages. Mary Norris's enthusiasm for the book's potential led to my contract with Globe Pequot. Mary nourished the book and me from start to publication with valuable contributions from editor Ellen Urban and graphic designers Diana Nuhn and Sheryl Kober.

Friends and family keep commitment alive over the years of development of a project like this. I particularly benefited from the insight, encouragement, and wise advice on an ongoing basis of Dr. Daniel Dachesky, Vassar classmates Judith Ehrlich and Betsy Barbanell, Robert Barbanell, Philippe Moussier, and Dr. Richard Taylor. Kevin Greenblat, Leslie Greenblat Shah, and Sachin Shah are a constant source of love and encouragement. My husband, John Gagnon, has provided inspiration in all my professional efforts, unflagging encouragement of my photographic endeavors, tolerance of my crazy work schedules, great cuisine, and much more—in short, quality caregiving in the fullest sense.

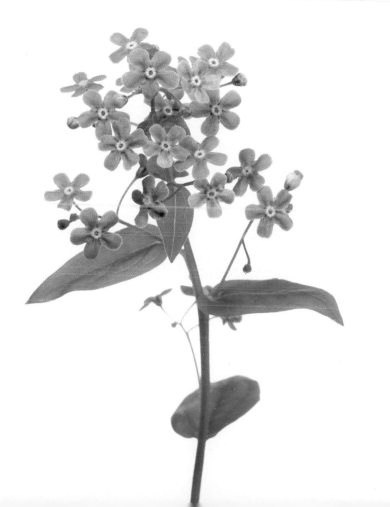

LOCATIONS

Canada – Baycrest Apotek Center, Toronto

Dominican Republic – home visits and visits to day- and residential-care programs in Santo Domingo

France – Center for Memory Resources and Research (CMRR), University Hospital Network (CHU) of Nice; Alzheimer's Côte d'Azur (ACA); Villa Helios, Nice; City of Nice program to welcome people with Alzheimer's to the museums; ARTZ (Artists for Alzheimer's) Paris

India – ARDSI (Alzheimer's and Related Disorders Society of India) programs in Cochin, Kunnamkulum, Delhi, Mumbai, and Bangalore; Nightingales' Foundation day program in Bangalore; home visits in Cochin, Delhi, and Mumbai

Japan – Several Rakuwakai group homes in Kyoto; Hajyodo Group Home in Nagoya; Uchida Hospital in Gunma province

Monaco – AMPA (Association Monégasque pour la Recherche sur la Maladie Alzheimer) program at the Speranza Center—Albert II Day Care Program

USA – Heather Hill Care Communities, Chardon, Ohio; The Intergenerational School, Cleveland, Ohio; four Silverado Senior Living Communities (Kingwood, Sugarland, Cypresswood, and Woodlands) in the Houston, Texas, area; Hearthstone at the Esplanade, New York City; Victoria Home, Montgomery Village, Maryland

RESOURCES

These are only a few of the many resources for your further exploration, but they are my favorites. More will be listed and updated regularly on the website for this book, www.lovelossandlaughter.com.

ADI (Alzheimer's Disease International). *World Alzheimer's Report 2009, World Alzheimer's Report 2010, World Alzheimer's Report 2011.* London: ADI, 2009 and 2010. Download at www.alz.co.uk/research/world-report.

Basting, Anne. *Forget Memory.* Baltimore: Johns Hopkins University Press, 2009.

Borrie, Cathie. *The Long Hello: The Other Side of Alzheimer's.* Vancouver: Nightwing Press, 2010.

Bryden, Christine. *Dancing with Dementia.* London: Jessica Kingsley Publishers, 2005.

Calkins, Margaret, et al. *Creating Successful Dementia Care Settings* (four-volume set). Baltimore: Health Professions Press, 2011.

Camp, Cameron. *Montessori Based Activities for Persons with Dementia.* Baltimore: Health Professions Press, 2001.

Cayton, Harry, Nori Graham, and James Warner. *Dementia: Alzheimer's and Other Dementias: The "At Your Fingertips" Guide.* London: Class Publishing, 2004.

Coste, Joanne Koenig. *Learning to Speak Alzheimer's.* Boston: Houghton Mifflin, 2003.

Doraiswamy, P. Murali, Lisa Gwyther, and Tina Adler. *The Alzheimer's Action Plan: The Experts' Guide to the Best Diagnosis and Treatment for Memory Problems.* New York: St. Martin's Press, 2008.

Fox, Judith. *"I Still Do."* New York: Powerhouse Books, 2009.

Genova, Lisa. *Still Alice.* Bloomington, IN: iUniverse Inc., 2007.

Greenblat, Cathy. *Alive with Alzheimer's.* Chicago: University of Chicago Press, 2004.

Guisset-Martinez, Marie-Jo, with Marion Villez. *Regaining Identity: New Synergies for a Different Approach to Alzheimer's: Guidelines for Professional Practices.* Paris: Fondation Médéric Alzheimer, 2011.

Kitwood, Tom. *Dementia Reconsidered: The Person Comes First.* Buckingham, UK, and Philadelphia: Open University Press, 1997.

Kuhn, Daniel. *Alzheimer's Early Stages: First Steps for Families, Friends and Caregivers.* Alameda, CA: Hunter House, second edition 2003; Kindle edition, 2011.

Mace, Nancy, and Peter Rabins. *The 36 Hour Day.* Baltimore: Johns Hopkins University Press, 2006.

Murray Alzheimer Research and Education (MAREP). "By Us for Us" guides. Free download at or purchase from MAREP, www.marep.uwaterloo.ca/products/bufu.html.

Power, Allen. *Dementia Beyond Drugs: Changing the Culture of Care.* Baltimore: Health Professions Press, 2010.

Rosenberg, Francesca, Amir Parsa, Laurel Humble, and Carrie McGee. *Meet Me: Making Art Accessible to People with Dementia.* Museum of Modern Art, 2009.

Shouse, Deborah. *Love in the Land of Dementia: Finding Hope in the Caregiver's Journey.* Kansas City, MO: Creation Connection Press, 2006.

Shriver, Maria. *The Shriver Report: A Woman's Nation Takes on Alzheimer's.* New York: Simon and Schuster, 2011.

———. *What's Happening to Grandpa?* Boston: Little, Brown, 2004.

Small, Neil, Katherine Froggatt, and Murna Downs. *Living and Dying with Dementia: Dialogues About Palliative Care.* New York: Oxford University Press, 2007.

Snyder, Lisa. *Living Your Best with Early-Stage Alzheimer's: An Essential Guide.* Northbranch, MN: Sunrise River Press, 2010.

Taylor, Richard. *Alzheimer's from the Inside Out.* Baltimore: Health Professions Press, 2007.

Whitehouse, Peter, and Daniel George. *The Myth of Alzheimer's.* Boston: Little, Brown, 2008.

Zeisel, John. *I'm Still Here.* New York: Penguin Group, 2009.

VIDEOS

Harrington, Eamon, and John Watkin. *Grandpa, Do You Know Who I Am?* The video can be seen online at www.hbo.com/alzheimers/grandpa-do-you-know-who-i-am.html.

Huebner, Berna, and Eric Ellena, *I Remember Better When I Paint . . .* Order from www.irememberbetterwhenipaint.com (available in English and in French).

Kashi, Ed, and Julie Winokur. *The Sandwich Generation.* Order from http://media storm.com/store/dvd-page/the-sandwich-generation.

Lichtenstein, Brad. *Almost Home.* Order from www.almosthomedoc.org.

Taylor, Richard. *Be with Me TODAY.* Order from www.richardtaylorphd.com.

Verde, Michael. *There Is a Bridge.* Order from www.memorybridge.org.

ABOUT THE AUTHOR

Cathy Greenblat, PhD (BA, Vassar College; MA, PhD Columbia University), has been engaged in a cross-cultural photographic project on aging, dementia, and end-of-life care since 2001. She is professor emerita of sociology at Rutgers University, where she served as a member of the Department of Sociology, Women's Studies, and the Bloustein School of Planning, teaching both undergraduate and graduate courses. During her academic career she authored more than a hundred professional articles and fourteen books. A photography-based book, *Alive with Alzheimer's*, and the German translation were published after her retirement.

Dr. Greenblat was based at Rutgers for most of her thirty-five-plus years of professional life, but she held visiting research and teaching appointments at the University of New Hampshire, Princeton University Graduate School of Arts and Sciences, Woodrow Wilson School of Public and International Affairs at Princeton, and Rutgers University Medical School (now UMDNJ). In addition, Professor Greenblat had short- and medium-term assignments from WHO, the World Bank, UNESCO, UNDP, IDRP, and other public agencies, and had committee or contract assignments from the Ford Foundation, the National Institutes of Health, the National Science Foundation, the Foundation for Science and Technology (Japan), the National Hemophilia Foundation, and other agencies and foundations.

Dr. Greenblat has lectured in the United States, Latin America, Eastern and Western Europe, Russia, Africa, India, the Philippines, China, and Japan. She was awarded the John P. McGovern, MD, Annual Award for work on Family, Health, and Human Values by the University of Houston in 2007 and delivered the 2010 Richard and Hinda Rosenthal Lecture at the Institute of Medicine. Photographs from this volume have been exhibited in the United States, Europe, and India. As the exhibits travel they will continue to heighten awareness and reduce stigma.

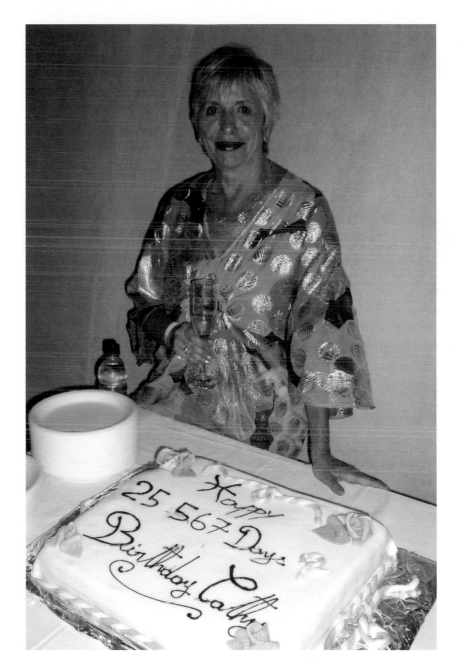

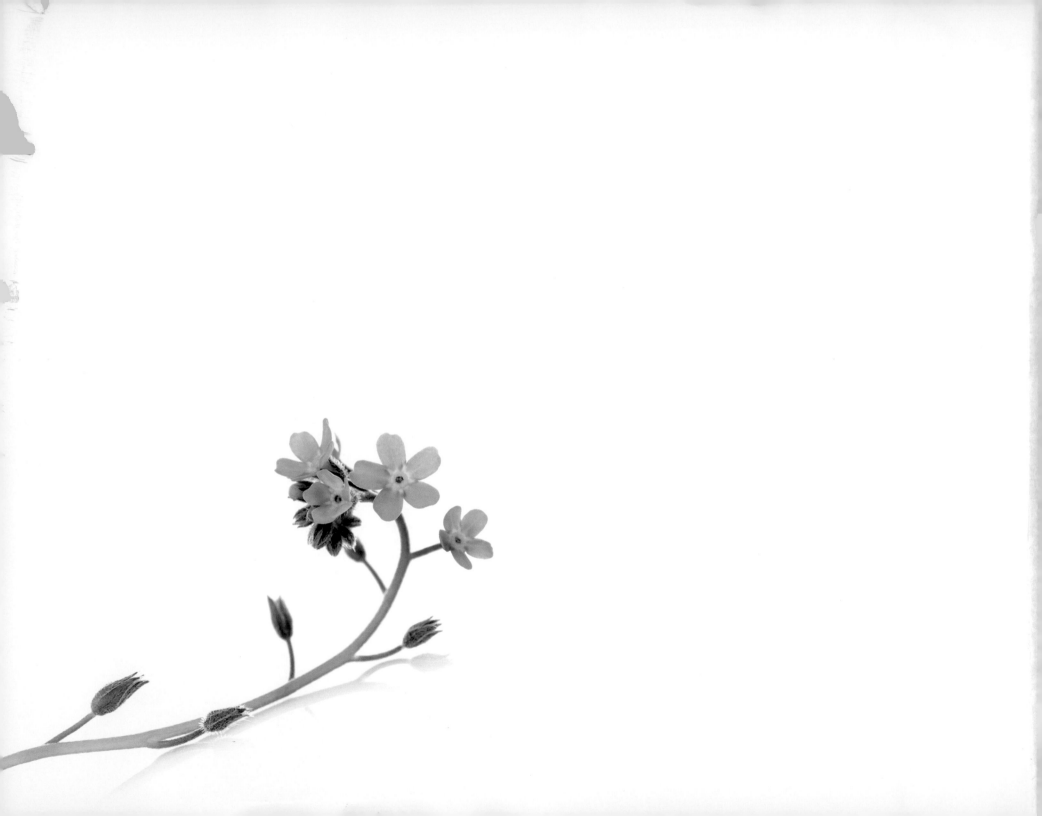